NEW ANESTHETIC AGENTS, DEVICES AND MONITORING TECHNIQUES

DEVELOPMENTS IN CRITICAL CARE MEDICINE AND ANAESTHESIOLOGY

Other volumes in this series:

Prakash, Omar (ed.): Applied Physiology in Clinical Respiratory Care. 1982. ISBN 90-247-2662-x.

McGeown, Mary G.: Clinical Management of Electrolyte Disorders. ISBN 90-247-2773-1.

Klain, Miroslav: High Frequency Ventilation.

Scheck, P.A.E., Smith, R. Brian and Sjöstrand, U: Perspectives in High Frequency Ventilation.

New Anesthetic Agents, Devices and Monitoring Techniques

Annual Utah Postgraduate Course in Anesthesiology 1983

edited by

THEODORE H. STANLEY, MD
W. CLAYTON PETTY, MD

Department of Anesthesiology
The University of Utah
Medical School
Salt Lake City, Utah 84132
USA

1983

MARTINUS NIJHOFF PUBLISHERS
BOSTON / THE HAGUE / DORDRECHT / LANCASTER

Distributors:

for the United States and Canada

Kluwer Boston, Inc.
190 Old Derby Street
Hingham, MA 02043
USA

for all other countries

Kluwer Academic Publishers Group
Distribution Center
P.O. Box 322
3300 AH Dordrecht
The Netherlands

Library of Congress Cataloging in Publication Data CIP

Main entry under title:

New anesthetic agents, devices, and monitoring techniques.

(Developments in critical care medicine and anesthesiology)
Includes bibliographical references.
1. Anesthetics--Addresses, essays, lectures.
2. Anesthesia--Addresses, essays, lectures.
3. Anesthesiology--Apparatus and instruments--Addresses, essays, lectures. I. Stanley, Theodore H.
II. Petty, W. Clayton. III. Series.
RD82.N48 1983 617'.96 82-22545

ISBN 90-247-2796-0

PRINTED IN THE USA

New Anesthetic Agents, Devices and Monitoring Techniques

Annual Utah Postgraduate Course in Anesthesiology 1983

edited by

THEODORE H. STANLEY, MD
W. CLAYTON PETTY, MD

Department of Anesthesiology
The University of Utah
Medical School
Salt Lake City, Utah 84132
USA

1983

MARTINUS NIJHOFF PUBLISHERS
BOSTON / THE HAGUE / DORDRECHT / LANCASTER

Distributors:

for the United States and Canada

Kluwer Boston, Inc.
190 Old Derby Street
Hingham, MA 02043
USA

for all other countries

Kluwer Academic Publishers Group
Distribution Center
P.O. Box 322
3300 AH Dordrecht
The Netherlands

Library of Congress Cataloging in Publication Data CIP

Main entry under title:

New anesthetic agents, devices, and monitoring techniques.

(Developments in critical care medicine and anesthesiology)
Includes bibliographical references.
1. Anesthetics--Addresses, essays, lectures.
2. Anesthesia--Addresses, essays, lectures.
3. Anesthesiology--Apparatus and instruments--Addresses, essays, lectures. I. Stanley, Theodore H.
II. Petty, W. Clayton. III. Series.
RD82.N48 1983 617'.96 82-22545

ISBN 90-247-2796-0

PRINTED IN THE USA

Contents

Contributing Authors vii

1. Current concepts in cerebral resuscitation/protection 1
J.D. Michenfelder, MD
2. Management of electrolyte abnormalities 10
K.C. Wong, MD, Ph.D.
3. Anesthetic management of the high risk pregnant patient: preeclampsia and diabetes 19
C.P. Gibbs, MD
4. Anesthesia for cerebral vascular surgery 45
J.D. Michenfelder, MD
5. Management of anesthesia in the presence of liver disease 48
R.K. Stoelting, MD
6. Special techniques in neuroanesthesia 55
J.D. Michenfelder, MD
7. Changing concepts in preanesthetic medication 60
R.K. Stoelting, MD
8. Calcium channel blockers and anesthesia 67
J.G. Reves
9. Comparisons between beta blockers and calcium entry blockers ... 77
J.H. Tinker, MD
10. Aspiration in obstetrics: etiology, prevention and treatment 83
C.P. Gibbs, MD
11. New developments in vasodilator therapy 92
J.H. Tinker, MD
12. Electrostimulation as an adjunct to anesthesia 98
T.H. Stanley, MD
13. New muscle relaxants 102
J.J. Savarese, MD
14. New intravenous anesthetic drugs: etomidate and midazolam 112
J.G. Reves
15. The new opioids 120
T.H. Stanley, MD
16. Comparative pharmacology of volatile anesthetics 127
R.K. Stoelting, MD
17. Prevention and treatment of intraoperative myocardial ischemia ... 134
J.H. Tinker, MD

18. Toxicity of local anesthetics in the adult, fetus and newborn 142
M. Finster, MD
19. Anesthesia for cesarean section: regional and general 147
C.P. Gibbs, MD
20. New aspects of nondepolarizing relaxant reversal 161
J.J. Savarese, MD
21. Buying a monitor 164
N.Ty Smith, MD
22. When are pulmonary artery catheters indicated in noncardiac surgery? 175
C.D. Blitt, MD
23. Monitoring the EEG in the operating room 179
N.Ty Smith, MD
24. Biochemical and biophysical monitoring of the fetus 188
M. Finster, MD
25. Are inhalation anesthetics better than injectable anesthetics for coronary artery surgery? 193
C.D. Blitt, MD
26. Continuous infusion of intravenous anesthetics: automated IV anesthesia, a rational method of drug administration 196
J.G. Reves, E.R. Greene, Jr., Th.N. Mackrell

Contributing Authors

Blitt, C.D., MD, Department of Anesthesiology, University of Arizona Health Sciences Center, Tucson AZ 85724, USA.

Finster, M., MD, Department of Anesthesiology, Columbia University College of Physicians and Surgeons, New York, NY 10032, USA.

Gibbs, C.P., MD, University of Florida, College of Medicine, Gainesville FL 32610, USA.

Greene, E.R., MD, University of Alabama in Birmingham, Department of Anesthesiology, Birmingham AL 35294, USA.

Mackrell, T.N., MD, University of Alabama in Birmingham, Department of Anesthesiology, Birmingham AL 35294, USA.

Michenfelder, J.D., MD, Department of Anesthesiology, Mayo Clinic, Rochester MN 55901, USA.

Pace, N.L., MD, University of Utah College of Medicine, Salt Lake City UT 84132, USA.

Petty, W.C., MD, The University of Utah, Medical School, Salt Lake City UT 84132, USA.

Reves, J.G., MD, University of Alabama in Birmingham, Department of Anesthesiology, Birmingham AL 35294, USA.

Savarese, J.J., MD, Massachusetts General Hospital, Department of Anesthesiology, Boston MA 02114, USA.

Smith, N.Ty, MD, University of California San Diego, Department of Anesthesiology, San Diego CA 92103, USA.

Stanley, T.H., MD, University of Utah School of Medicine, Department of Anesthesiology, Salt Lake City, UT 84132, USA.

Stoelting, R.K., MD, Indiana University School of Medicine, Department of Anesthesiology, Indianapolis, IN 46223, USA.

Tinker, J.H., MD, Mayo Clinic, Department of Anesthesiology, Rochester, MN 55905, USA.

Wong, K.C., MD, Ph D, University of Utah School of Medicine, Department of Anesthesiology, Salt Lake City, UT 84132, USA.

NEW ANESTHETIC AGENTS, DEVICES AND MONITORING TECHNIQUES

NEW ANESTHETIC AGENTS, DEVICES AND MONITORING TECHNIQUES

1
CURRENT CONCEPTS IN CEREBRAL RESUSCITATION/PROTECTION

J.D. MICHENFELDER, M.D.

Prior to 1950 it was commonly assumed that cerebral injury resulting from such events as cardiac arrest, stroke, or head trauma was nearly immediate in onset and irreversible. Post-injury therapy was supportive only. In the past 30 years intermittent enthusiasm has emerged for various interventions which appeared promising in animal studies but failed in clinical trials. In the mid-1950's hypothermia was viewed as a major step forward in cerebral resuscitation. However, after an initial wave of enthusiasm, the use of hypothermia was largely abandoned presumably because of either unfavorable experience or at least unconvincing evidence that the benefits in any way justified the complexity, risk, and expense of prolonged hypothermia. In the early 1970's enthusiasm waxed for the use of hyperventilation in at least some of these patients but this too was largely abandoned (except for head trauma patients) in a few years again for presumably the same reasons. Steroid therapy has also enjoyed varying degrees of enthusiasm during this period and although still controversial, it remains in common use largely because of a very low risk-benefit ratio.

BARBITURATES

In the late 1970's barbiturate therapy achieved a status comparable to that once enjoyed by hypothermia and hyperventilation. Although too early to pass judgement, there is a growing impression that enthusiasm for this mode of therapy is now also on the wane. If this impression is correct, then it is tempting to conclude that the carefully controlled animal models used in past years to demonstrate efficacy for various modes of therapy cannot be considered analgous to the clinical circumstances confronted following cardiac arrest, stroke or head trauma. Rather, it would seem that these clinical conditions present a heterogeneous cerebral and systemic pathologic state which in total is not favorably affected by such interventions. It should be noted that for each mode of therapy (hypothermia, hyperventilation, barbiturate therapy) no controlled clinical trials have ever been completed which permit an objective evaluation of efficacy. This in large part reflects the heterogeneous nature of the pathologic states such that it is not possible to create matched control and treatment groups nor is it possible to blind the observer to the nature of the intervention.

Although the above would appear to be a pessimistic evaluation, much useful information has been uncovered in efforts to develop clinically useful techniques of cerebral resuscitation. Thus although it was once thought that the brain could not recover from more than a 4-5 minute period of circulatory arrest, there is now both anecdotal evidence in man and experimental evidence in animals that, under proper circumstances, the brain's tolerance to total ischemia can apparently be extended. The precise nature of these modifying circumstances are as yet, however, not well defined.

We know from animal models that following a period of circulatory arrest, there is a brief period of reactive hyperemia (20-30 minutes) followed by a prolonged period of a severe hypoperfusion state which may or may not be associated with areas of no-reflow.[1,2] The cause of this hypoperfusion state remains unknown but preliminary animal work indicates that calcium entry blockers might favorably affect this hypoperfusion state. On the assumption that this prolonged period of hypoperfusion contributes to the ultimate brain damage, there is reason to believe that appropriate intervention once identified might significantly alter the outcome following cardiac arrest. In this regard, it should be noted that those studies[3,4] which suggest that a state of very low cerebral blood flow (less than 10% of normal) is more damaging to the brain than no flow at all are based upon metabolic and electrophysiologic observations only and not upon meaningful cerebral functional evaluation. A recent study[5] which examined for such function yielded the reassuring results that some blood flow, no matter how small, is better than no flow at all in terms of cerebral function recovery.

If barbiturates can play a favorable role in the post-cardiac arrest period, the mechanism for such an effect has not been uncovered. To date, the experimental evidence for such a beneficial effect is contradictory[6-10] (Table) such that only two of six animal studies have reported any degree of functional improvement when barbiturates were given either before or after a period of complete global ischemia. Clinical evidence for a beneficial effect is both contradictory and anecdotal only. It is, however, generally agreed that if barbiturates are beneficial this effect must be unrelated to any effect on either cerebral metabolism or intracranial pressure. That barbiturates might act by scavenging free radicals formed during and following the period of resuscitation is an appealing theory which, however, has not stood up to experimental evaluation.[11,12] At this point a very cautious and skeptical attitude towards the use of barbiturates following cardiac arrest would appear appropriate. Recommendations must await further investigational work.

In stroke patients the use of barbiturate therapy cannot be recommended at this time despite the fact that stroke models in laboratory animals have been shown consistently to be benefited by administration of barbiturates either before or after initiation of the stroke.[13,14] Clearly the lesion resulting from the abrupt occlusion of a single cerebral vessel in an otherwise healthy animal cannot be equated to that encountered in the stroke patient. The latter is usually aged with diffuse cerebrovascular disease and commonly has accompanying severe systemic pathology (cardiac and renal primarily). In such patients to induce prolonged deep barbiturate coma must be considered a high risk venture which is difficult to justify.

Still there are useful clinical applications for barbiturate therapy in circumstances analagous to the animal stroke models which have been investigated. Thus in intraoperative situations where it is necessary to temporarily occlude a major extracranial or intracranial vessel (for example, carotid endarterectomy; bypass procedures; aneurysm surgery) or in circumstances where profound degrees of hypotension are required, barbiturate therapy may well be indicated and might reasonably be expected to prolong the brain's tolerance to any induced ischemia. Lacking evidence to the contrary, it is reasonable to assume that the magnitude of the protection is directly related to the magnitude of metabolic depression induced by the barbiturate. Hence, the dose of barbiturate should be that which would nearly completely suppress the EEG. This is similar to a "sleep dose" of thiopental or approximately 3-5 mg/kg. In these intraoperative circumstances the risk-benefit ratio is relatively low since the patient is already anesthetized and adequate monitoring is ongoing.

It has also been learned from animal stroke models that the brain does not immediately infarct following occlusion of a single major vessel but rather irreversible damage may not occur for as long as 2-3 hours[15] (depending upon collateral flow). This gives hope for the future that an appropriate intervention will be identified which can be initiated during this potentially reversible period. From a surgical standpoint this also means that acute vascular occlusions should be corrected if technically possible as soon as recognized (even if as long as 3-4 hours following the event).

Perhaps the greatest progress has been made clinically in the management of head trauma patients. This is particularly so in those centers that have adopted an aggressive attitude toward the management of these patients. Success is in part accounted for by the fact that, as compared to stroke and cardiac arrest patients, the average age of the head trauma patients is much younger. The introduction of routine monitoring of intracranial pressure (ICP) represents a major step forward in the management of these patients. It is this monitor which provides the primary guide for the mode and magnitude of therapy used. Thus in the presence of an elevated ICP, administration of hyperosmotic agents and the use of hyperventilation represent routine interventions that often result in control of ICP. Although controversial, many also routinely use large doses of steroids in head trauma patients. Because of the low-risk benefit ratio this may be reasonable even though the results in clinical trials are contradictory.

In patients with elevated ICP that is refractory to routine interventions, the use of barbiturate therapy has once again been recommended. In this instance, the recommendation is not primarily based upon some hoped for "protective" effect, but rather it is based on the well recognized potential for barbiturates to reduce intracranial pressure, presumably by reducing cerebral blood flow concomitant with the reduction in cerebral metabolism. In the first large series reported[16] using this mode of therapy the results appeared most promising and suggested that some 25 percent of head trauma patients fall into the category of those who would benefit from barbiturate therapy. However, it should be noted that in an even larger reported series[17] of head trauma patients, the overall morbidity and mortality was the same without the use of barbiturates. Thus, although barbiturates are clearly effective in reducing ICP, it remains uncertain whether their use does in fact improve prognosis as compared to those patients treated aggressively with steroids, hyperosmotic agents and hyperventilation. It should be noted that barbiturates have also been recommended for the treatment of Reye's syndrome, again for elevated ICP which is refractory to standard therapy. However, as with head trauma patients, others have reported equally good results in the treatment of Reye's syndrome without barbiturate therapy[18].

After reviewing the above, it would seem apparent that barbiturate therapy is not a panacea and that the indications for clinical application are at best confused. We know that barbiturates significantly reduce cerebral metabolic rate, significantly reduce cerebral blood flow, and because of the latter effect, have the potential to significantly reduce ICP. The ability to abruptly reduce cerebral metabolic demands may be clinically useful in those limited circumstances where an acute reduction in cerebral blood flow is unavoidable. The ability to reduce ICP may be useful in those patients in whom routine therapy is ineffective in accomplishing this goal. Outside of these two quite limited indications, a skeptical attitude would seem warranted regarding barbiturate therapy for brain damaged patients.

EVALUATION OF OTHER POTENTIAL PROTECTIVE DRUGS

In addition to barbiturates there are a number of other therapeutic interventions that have been suggested as being possibly either protective or ameliorative whether given before or after a period of complete global ischemia. Gamma-hydroxybutyrate was previously reported in rats to reduce cerebral metabolic rate to as low as 35 percent of control and was therefore suggested as being a perhaps potent protective agent.[19] In dogs gamma-hydroxybutyrate reduced cerebral metabolic rate to about 60 percent of control but at the same time cerebral blood flow was reduced to less than 50 percent of control.[20] Thus the ratio of flow to metabolic rate was unfavorably altered. When tested in the hypoxic mouse model, gamma-hydroxybutyrate was found to increase survival time (less than two-fold) but to a much lesser degree than that provided by barbiturate therapy (about four-fold). Thus it would appear that the unfavorable effects of gamma-hydroxybutyrate on cerebral blood flow limit the degree of protection provided by the metabolic depression in the hypoxic mouse model.

Phenytoin has been reported in a number of different animal models to provide a degree of cerebral protection. The mechanism for such an effect has not been established. In dogs even large doses of phenytoin had essentially no effect on cerebral metabolic rate and resulted in only a modest decrease in cerebral blood flow.[21] Yet in the hypoxic mouse model a more than two-fold degree of protection was provided (more than gamma-hydroxybutyrate but less than barbiturates) which cannot be explained by either a metabolic or cerebral blood flow effect. Others have observed that phenytoin decreases the release of potassium from ischemic neurons and glial cells as reflected by the rate of accumulation of potassium in cerebral spinal fluid. This presumably relates to the membrane stabilization effects of phenytoin and possibly accounts for any protection since it has been postulated that release of potassium contributes to the irreversible neuronal damage that occurs during and following ischemia.

Midazolam is a new water soluble benzodiazepine which is being recommended as an induction agent for anesthesia. In the dog it is a potent depressant of cerebral metabolic rate, similar to that observed with thiopental. Like thiopental, it does not unfavorably alter the ratio between cerebral blood flow and cerebral metabolism. In addition systemic hemodynamic depression is not a major feature of midazolam induced anesthesia. In the hypoxic mouse model midazolam was found to provide a significant degree of protection (about three-fold; greater than phenytoin but less than pentobarbital). This suggests that midazolam, because of less systemic hemodynamic depression, may prove to be a useful agent for the purposes of brain protection.

Isoflurane also appears to offer unique promise for potential brain protection. It is the only inhalational agent that can produce an isoelectric EEG at concentrations that are hemodynamically tolerated. Both in man and dogs this occurs at about 2 MAC. In dogs this is associated with a 60% reduction in $CMRO_2$ (the same as maximal depression with thiopental) and no evidence of toxicity (unlike halothane). In a canine model of hemorrhagic hypotension isoflurane was found to protect the brain to the same degree as did thiopental and in the hypoxic mouse model isoflurane also provided protection. Thus isoflurane possibly offers a means of providing protection comparable to that provided by barbiturates without the same degree of hemodynamic depression and with the ability to rapidly reverse this effect when protection is no longer required.

HYPOTHERMIA

The role of hypothermia in brain resuscitation remains controversial There would seem to be no reason to question that acute hypothermia will significantly prolong the brain's tolerance for varying periods of ischemia depending upon the degree of hypothermia. Whether or not hypothermia induced after a period of complete global ischemia offers any beneficial effects remains unknown.

There is reason to believe that prolonged hypothermia (1-3 days) introduces complications that are not apparent when hypothermia is used for acute purposes only (that is of several hours duration). When cats are cooled to 29°C for 48 hours and then rewarmed by external means there consistently develops a severe systemic acidosis followed by hemodynamic collapse and death.[22] In dogs cooling to 29°C produces the expected

immediate 50 percent reduction in cardiac output and wholebody oxygen consumption.[23] However, with continued maintenance of hypothermia at 29°C there is a progressive reduction in both cardiac output and oxygen consumption such that after 24 hours cardiac output is on the average less than 10 percent of control whereas oxygen consumption is reduced to about 30 percent of control. At this point, however, acid-base balance and vital signs appear normal. With rewarming cardiac output fails to increase significantly, oxygen consumption increases only moderately and a severe acidosis develops with hemodynamic collapse. In both dogs and cats following 24-48 hours of hypothermia (29°C) there develops a striking degree of heterogeneous perfusion, particularly in skeletal muscle, as evaluated by post-mortem carbon black injections. In the normothermic animal, carbon black deeply stains all of the tissues of the body whereas in animals maintained hypothermic for 24-48 hours, there are, throughout the body, large areas of muscle that are unstained by carbon black. Similarly in the cortex of the brain of both monkeys and dogs following 24-48 hours of hypothermia there can be identified areas of very low or no flow. Thus it would appear that the maintenance of normal vital signs and a normal acid-base balance during prolonged hypothermia is accounted for by a significant increase in peripheral vascular resistance with shutdown of many vascular beds which then trap accumulating acid metabolites. With rewarming some of these vascular beds presumably reopen which results in a flooding of the systemic circulation with acid metabolites and hemodynamic collapse.

Whether or not these effects of chronic hypothermia are operative in man remains unknown. But there are suggestions that such may occur. In reviewing the older hypothermia literature, one finds the term "rewarming shock" as part of the hypothermia lexicon; although, no mechanisms were identified. In the original description of the use of prolonged moderate hypothermia by Fay (for the treatment of metastatic carcinoma) there was an overall mortality in 124 patients of 15 percent.[24] Of the 19 patients that died only two died during hypothermia, the remainder died during or shortly following rewarming. In an unpublished series of 12 stroke patients cooled for several days to 29°C, 10 of the 12 patients died upon rewarming.[25] Finally as noted in the introduction, the fact that chronic hypothermia was largely discarded in the late 50's and early 60's after an enthusiastic reception suggests that, despite the theoretical benefits there were in fact unexpected complications of an unspecified nature.

CONCLUSION

In summary, specific therapeutic intervention for cerebral resuscitation following cardiac arrest remains controversial. Those interventions which introduce additional risks for patients already in a precarious state should be rigorously demonstrated to be effective in valid animal models before applied clinically. An overview of the past 30 years suggests that "fads" rather than "facts" have had an overwhelming influence upon well meaning but often poorly informed clinicians who are anxious to offer some hope in a clinical situation that is often simply hopeless. The temptation to introduce such well intended interventions can be resisted by examining available lessons from the recent past.

BARBITURATE PROTECTION/AMELIORATION IN GLOBAL BRAIN ANOXIA

(Functional Studies Only)

Investigator	Year	Species	Anoxia	Barb.	Prot./ Amel
Goldstein, et al	1966	Dog	Vessel lig.	Pent (pre)	Yes
Bleyaert, et al	1978	Primate	Choke	Thio (post)	Yes
Steen, et al	1979	Dog	Vessel lig.	Pent (pre)	No
Snyder, et al	1979	Dog	Asphyxia	Thio (post)	No
Chadwick, et al	1980(abs)	Cat	Fibrillation	Thio (post)	No
Gisvold, et al	1981(abs)	Primate	Choke	Thio (post)	No

REFERENCES

1. Steen PA, Milde JH, Michenfelder JD: Cerebral metabolic and vascular effects of barbiturate therapy following complete global ischemia. J Neurochem 31:1317-1324, 1978.
2. Snyder JV, Nemoto EM, Carroll RG: Global ischemia in dogs: Intracranial pressures, brain blood flow and metabolism. Stroke 6:21-27, 1975.
3. Siesjo BK, Nordstrom C-H, Rehncrona S: Metabolic aspects of cerebral hypoxia-ischemia. Adv Exp Med Biol 78:261-269, 1977.
4. Hossman K-A, Kleihues P: Reversibility of ischemic brain damage. Arch Neurol 29:375-384, 1973.
5. Steen PA, Michenfelder JD, Milde JH: Incomplete versus complete cerebral ischemia: Improved outcome with a minimal blood flow. Ann Neurol 6: 389-398, 1979.
6. Goldstein A Jr, Wells BA, Keats AS: Increased tolerance to cerebral anoxia by pentobarbital. Arch Int Pharmacodyn 161:138-143, 1966.
7. Bleyaert A, Nemoto EM, Safar P, et al: Thiopental amelioration of brain damage after global ischemia in monkeys. Anesthesiology 49:390-398, 1978.
8. Steen PA, Milde JH, Michenfelder JD: No barbiturate protection in a dog model of complete cerebral ischemia. Ann Neurol 5:343-349, 1979.
9. Snyder BD, Raminez-Lassepas M, Sukhum P, et al: Failure of thiopental to modify global anoxia. Stroke 10:135-141, 1979.

10. Chadwick HS, Todd MM, Shapiro HM, et al: Neurologic outcome following cardiac arrest in thiopental treated cats. Anesthesiology 53:S156, 1980.
11. Steen PA, Michenfelder JD: Cerebral protection with barbiturates. Relation to anesthetic effect. Stroke 9:140-142, 1978.
12. Smith DS, Rehncrona S, Siesjo BK: Inhibitory effects of different barbiturates of lipid peroxidation in brain tissue in vitro: Comparison with the effects of promethaxine and chlorpormaxine. Anesthesiology 53:186-194, 1980.
13. Smith AL, Hoff JT, Nielsen SL, et al: Barbiturate protection in acute focal cerebral ischemia. Stroke 5:1-7, 1974.
14. Michenfelder JD, Milde JH, Sundt TM Jr: Cerebral Protection by barbiturate anesthesia. Arch Neurol 33:345-350, 1976.
15. Sundt TM Jr, Grant WC, Carcia JH: Restoration of middle cerebral artery flow in experimental infarction. J Neurosurg 31:311-326, 1969.
16. Marshall LF, Smith RW, Shapiro HM: The outcome with aggressive treatment in severe head injuries: I. The significance of intracranial pressure monitoring; II. Acute and chronic barbiturate administration in the management of head injury. J Neurosurg 50:20-30, 1979.
17. Miller JD: Barbiturates and raised intracranial pressure. Ann Neurol 6:189-193, 1979.
18. Trauner DA: Treatment of Reye Syndrome. Ann Neurol 7:2-4, 1980.
19. Wolfson LI, Sakurado O, Sokoloff L: Effects of γ-butyrolactone on local cerebral glucose utilization in the rat. J Neurochem 29:777-783, 1980.
20. Artru AA, Steen PA, Michenfelder JD: γ-Hydroxybutyrate: Cerebral metabolic, vascular, and protective effects. J Neurochem 35:1114-1119, 1980.
21. Artru AA, Michenfelder JD: Cerebral protective, metabolic and vascular effects of phenytoin. Stroke 11:377-382, 1980.
22. Steen PA, Soule EH, Michenfelder JD: Detrimental effect of prolonged hypothermia in cats and monkeys with and without regional cerebral ischemia. Stroke 10:522-529, 1979
23. Steen PA, Milde JH, Michenfelder JD: The detrimental effects of prolonged hypothermia and rewarming in the dog. Anesthesiology 52: 224-230, 1980.
24. Fay T: Early experiences with local and generalized refrigeration of the human brain. J Neurosurg 16:239-260, 1959.
25. Field WS: Houston, Texas. Personal communication.

MANAGEMENT OF ELECTROLYTE ABNORMALITIES

K. C. WONG, M.D., Ph.D.

Proper distribution of cations between the intracellular and extracellular space is essential for maintaining homeostasis. Potassium is important for maintaining resting membrane potential and repolarization of excitable cells. Proper sodium concentration in the extracellular space is essential for depolarization, the production of action potentials of excitable cells, and for its osmotic effect in the extracellular fluid. Calcium sets the threshold of excitation and is necessary for muscle contraction. Magnesium is an important cation for a variety of cellular functions and is a potent neurodepressant when administered in therapeutic amounts for treatment of toxemia of pregnancy. This review considers some pertinent aspects of electrophysiology which are influenced by changes in concentration of potassium, sodium, calcium, and magnesium; and discusses clinical situations during which these cations can influence the anesthetic management of the patient.

Endogenous Cations and Electrophysiology of Cardiac Cell

Potassium is the predominant intracellular cation, while sodium is the predominant extracellular cation. The electrolyte solutions of both inside and outside the cell contain about 155 mEq/L of cations and anions. The ionic distributions and concentration gradients between the intra- and extra-cellular compartments are responsible for generating electrical potentials of mammalian cells for exerting appropriate physiologic functions of the cells. The approximate steady-state ionic concentrations and the electrical potential they generate in mammalian muscle cells and interstitial fluid are shown in the Table.

The resting membrane potential of about -90 mV, inside with respect to the outside of cardiac cells, is primarily produced by the transmembrane potassium concentration gradient. Mathematically, the Nernst equation is useful for estimating the resting membrane potential.

$$E = 60 \log_{10} \frac{[K]o}{[K]i}$$

$$E = 60 \log_{10} \frac{4}{155}$$

$$E = -90 \text{ mV}$$

The excitable cell generates an action potential (electrical signal) when its threshold of excitation is reached. The "sodium gate" opens and depolarization occurs by an inrushing of sodium ions through "fast channels," into the cell, thus producing an action potential. The threshold of excitation can be elicited by an electrical, chemical or mechanical stimulus. In the case of the sinoatrial node of the myocardium, there is spontaneous depolarization from influx of calcium through "slow channels" into the cell until the threshold is reached. (Automaticity describes such cells which displays spontaneous depolarization.) The resting membrane potential is, therefore, important for governing cardiac excitability and generating an effective action potential. The action potential of the sinoatrial node is helpful to illustrate these electrophysiological principles (Figure 1) which are applicable to all excitable cells.

Repolarization of the cardiac cell is also an important function of the transmembrane potassium concentration gradient, since it is the immediate movement of K^+ out of the cell that repolarizes the cardiac cell. The Na-K pump, then, serves as a physiological "generator" to pump K^+ into and Na^+ out of the cardiac cell thus maintaining the proper electrolytic gradients. The ECG manifestations of hypokalemia and hyperkalemia are depicted in the Figure.

Calcium and magnesium are also important for controlling cardiac excitability. Calcium binds negative sites in the channels for Na^+, thus setting the level of threshold for excitation (opening the sodium gate). Hypercalcemia elevates the threshold for maximal Na^+ permeability while hypocalcium lowers the threshold. Magnesium may control calcium ion movements and distribution in several types of muscles, thus also regulate cardiac excitability. High extracellular concentrations of magnesium depress atrioventricular and intraventricular conduction, while hypomagnesemia can produce cardiac arrhythmias including ventricular fibrillation and sudden asystole.

Potassium

Hypokalemia is, by definition, a reduction in serum potassium concentration. Clinically the only practical means of assessing electrolyte disturbances of the body is by measurement of serum concentrations. However, serum $[K^+]$ normally represents only 1/39 of intracellular $[K^+]$ (Table 1). Therefore, it is important to distinguish acute hypokalemia, a reduction of serum $[K^+]$ without loss of total body potassium, from chronic hypokalemia, a reduction of serum $[K^+]$ with loss of total body potassium.

Acute hypokalemia can be induced by transmembrane movement of extracellular K^+ into cells in exchange for intracellular H^+ as a means of physiologic compensation for acute serum alkalemia. Acute serum acidemia causes shifts in the opposite direction. When acid-base disturbances is chronic, renal mechanisms become more important for maintaining acid-base balance in the body. Acute hypokalemia is a common iatrogenic product of hyperventilation during anesthesia and is not a problem in an ASA Class I patient. It is estimated that for every 0.1 pH unit increase, there could be an 0.5-1.0 mEq/L K^+ shift into the intracellular compartment.

Chronic hypokalemia is detrimental to cardiac function. Some common causes of potassium loss are diarrhea, nasogastric suction, hyperaldosteronism, digitalis and diuretic therapy. Hypokalemia from digitalis and/or diuretic therapy is the most common type of potassium-deficient surgical patient, and perhaps one of the most difficult patients for anesthetic management. Indeed, these patients usually have significant cardiovascular disease (i.e. cardiac failure, atherosclerosis, hypertension and myocardial ischemic disease). Many chronic hypokalemic patients (serum $[K^+]$ below 3.0 mEq/L, do not manifest cardiac arrhythmias except for low T-waves on the ECG, suggesting the importance of potassium gradient across the cell membrane for maintaining cardiac stability. On the other hand, the heart of potassium-depleted patients is less capable of maintaining homeostasis when challenged by surgery, anesthesia, acid-base imbalance and stress. The more profound is the chronic hypokalemia, the greater is the propensity to develop dangerous cardiac arrhythmias. To confuse the matter, there is evidence to suggest that cellular potassium loss may not be reflected by serum [K^+]. Patients, receiving K^+ losing diuretics, with metabolic alkalosis and normokalemia, having "therapeutic" concentrations of digoxin, had significantly greater cardiac arrhythmias than did patients without alkalosis. In addition to the electrophysiologic disturbance created by potassium imbalance, intracellular potassium deficit is also associated with poor cardiac contractility. Chronic hypokalemia has been blamed for unsuccessful cardiopulmonary resuscitations and unexplained cardiac arrests. Unfortunately, there are no good published data to substantiate this clinical impression.

Potassium Therapy

Serum potassium concentration alone is not a reliable reflection of total body [K^+]. With the aid of a good history and physical, ECG and objective measurements of potassium loss (e.g. urinary excretion during cardiopulmonary bypass and serum potassium measurements), one can administer potassium more rationally.

The degree of chronic potassium loss, magnitude of contemplated surgery, physical status of the patient and skills of the surgeon and anesthesiologist are all important factors for assessing the surgical risk of the patient. Thus, it is generally agreed that a chronic hypokalemic patient with a serum [K^+] of 3.0 mEq/L is the minimal acceptable level for elective surgery and 3.5 mEq/L is the minimal acceptable level in a digitalized patient.

A 25% reduction of body potassium may exceed 1000 mEq. Theoretically, at least 6-10 days would be required for repletion of such magnitude of potassium deficit based upon a maximal recommended dose of 240 mEq/day and a daily obligatory loss of 50-100 mEq. One cannot expect, then, to replete such deficits by rapid intravenous administration of KCl. In fact rapid IV administration of KCl in experimental animals is rapidly excreted by the kidneys without significant retention of K^+ by the body. However, there are published data to suggest that IV KCl may exert an antiarrhythmic effect in the potassium-depleted patient, especially if the patient is also digitalized.

Guidelines for Potassium Administration

1. When time permits, oral potassium 25 mEq every 6-8 hours for one week is the safest and perhaps the most effective way of replenishing body potassium.
2. Intravenous KCl is limited to 0.5 mEq/kg/hr.
3. Do not exceed 240 mEq/24 hr.
4. Monitor the ECG and serum electrolyte.
5. When emergency surgery does not allow at least 12 hours for potassium administration, 0.5 mEq/kg/hr of KCl in 10% dextrose is helpful to facilitate cellular uptake of potassium.
6. Avoid iatrogenic acid-base disturbance.

Acute hyperkalemia is the result of a sudden increase in serum [K^+] and can cause a reduction (more positive) in resting membrane potential with an increase in cardiac excitability. Further increases in serum [K^+] will produce conduction block from poor depolarization and repolarization and finally persistent membrane depolarization and cardiac arrest (Figure 1). An important consideration of acute hyperkalemia during anesthesia is the use of succinylcholine in severely burned, traumatized, or cord-injured patients. The most reliable indices for predicting a dangerous increase in serum potassium following intravenous administration of succinylcholine were shown to be 1) the time elapsed from burn injury to anesthesia and 2) the extent of the burn injury. However, hyperkalemia due to succinylcholine administration was evident as early as nine days following injury, and increases in serum potassium to more than 6 mEq/L were observed in patients with total burned surfaces of as little as 8% (i.e. less than the surface of one arm). This K^+-releasing effect begins 5-15 days after injury. It persists for 60-90 days after thermal and crushing injuries, and at least 3-6 months after upper-motor-neuron lesions. There is some question as to whether succinylcholine should ever be used in the presence of chronic, wasting neuromuscular blocking agent prior to succinylcholine cannot be depended upon to prevent hyperkalemia following succinylcholine in burned patients.

Chronic hyperkalemia implies a gradual increase in extracellular $[K^+]$ with or without a simultaneous increase in intracellular $[K^+]$. This condition commonly exists in chronic renal failure. The fact that these patients generally tolerate serum potassium levels in excess of 6 mEq/L without apparent cardiovascular symptoms supports the importance of an appropriate $[K^+]$ gradient rather than the concentration of K^+ per se across the cell membrane.

Uremic patients needing hemodialysis usually have other concomitant electrolytic disturbances: 1) hyponatremia; 2) hypermagnesemia; 3) hypocalcemia. The major pharmacologic actions of magnesium are vasodilation, central nervous system depression, and neuromuscular blockade. The net effect of these electrolytic disturbances in uremic patients renders them more sensitive to nervous system depressants (i.e. they need less CNS depressants and neuromuscular blocking agents).

Hyperkalemia, however, has the most detrimental effect on myocardial electrical activity. When cardiac function is impaired, treatment of hyperkalemia should include:

1. Monitoring the ECG and serum electrolytes.
2. Intravenous administration of calcium to restore the balance between K^+ and Ca^{++} (as an acute emergency measure by continuous infusion until the sine wave reverts to a normal ECG complex; then rapidly institute other means).
3. Lowering serum K^+
   a. $NaHCO_3$ infusion when hyperkalemia is accompanied by acidosis; the severity of acidosis should be determined by blood-gas measurements.
   b. Administration of glucose plus insulin increases cellular uptake of K^+; this is given as a 25% solution with 0.5 unit of regular insulin for each 2 g glucose -- as much as 300 ml of glucose may be given in 30 minutes.
   c. Cation exchange resin by mouth or rectum, usually 20-50 g/day.
   d. Hemodialysis.

Sodium

Sodium imbalance is usually associated with potassium imbalance. Sodium, in addition to being important for the depolarization of excitable cells, is also important for its osmotic effect in the extracellular fluid.

Hyponatremia, in the presence of a decreased extracellular fluid volume, is encountered when body fluids containing electrolytes which are lost are replaced with electrolyte-free solutions. Hyponatremia accompanied by an increased decompensation, in hepatic cirrhosis with ascites, or in the nephrotic syndrome. Restriction of sodium intake, while allowing a free fluid intake, contributes to the problem of hyponatremia with edema. The condition of these patients is frequently refractory to diuretics until electrolyte balance has been restored. Poor cardiac performance and increased sensitivity to nondepolarizing neuromuscular blocking agents are to be expected in these patients. A serious intraoperative complication is dilutional hyponatremia secondary to absorption of irrigating fluid during transurethral resection.

The symptoms of dilutional hyponatremia include:

1. With regional anesthesia, restlessness is an early symptom and may be associated with irritability and confusion. A serum [Na^+] of 120 mEq/L appears to be borderline between mild and severe reactions.
2. Hypotension and tachycardia.
3. ECG changes characterized by widening of the QRS complex and ST segment elevation when [Na^+] falls to 115 mEq/L (approx.).
4. Seizures occur at serum [Na^+] 102 mEq/L (approx.).
5. Ventricular tachycardia or fibrillation may occur at serum [Na^+] 100 mEq/L or less.

Principles of treatment of hyponatremia include:

1. Successful treatment depends upon early detection.
2. Termination of the surgical procedure and anesthesia usually results in prompt diuresis.
3. When cardiovascular embarrassment exists, the administration of sodium chloride (NaCl), diuretics and vasoactive agents may be helpful.
4. Serial monitoring and serum electrolytes.

Hypernatremia is usually the result of excessive free-water clearance with inadequate intake. Diabetes insipidus due to head injury is frequently accompanied by hypernatremia and a clouded sensorium. Chronic steroid therapy is associated with hypernatremia and hypokalemia.

Calcium

Endogenous hyper- and hypocalcemia are usually due to various well-known endocrine disorders. Hypercalcemic nephropathy and hypocalcemic tetany are also well-known clinical entities. Hypercalcemia increases the threshold of excitation and hypocalcemia lowers the threshold. Ionized calcium is the active form and is pH-dependent; thus, alkalosis can reduce serum [Ca^{++}] as well as serum [K^+].

The plasma of acid-citrate-dextrose (ACD) blood stored at 4° C has been shown to gain about 1 mEq/L K^+/unit blood/day, increased to 32 mEq/L after 21 days of storage. Most of the K^+ re-enters the erythrocytes after transfusion and, in some cases, hypokalemia is observed. The pH steadily decreases to approximately 6.5 after 21 days because of cellular metabolism and the formation of lactic and pyruvic acids. Hypothermia from rapid administration of cold blood can enhance acidosis and myocardial depression. Citrate intoxication is characterized by hypotension, a narrowed pulse pressure, and elevated left ventricular end-diastolic and central venous pressures. Binding of ionized calcium by the citrate in ACD solution can produce myocardial depression. Hepatic disease tends to reduce the metabolism of citrate and enhance its toxicity.

Cardiac contractility is closely dependent upon extracellular calcium concentration. Extracellular calcium is in equilibrium with the mobile fraction of intracellular calcium. Calcium binds the troponin complex in muscle, which normally inhibits cross-bridge formation between actin and myosin, thus producing muscle contraction. The sarcoplasmic reticulum reversibly binds calcium to produce relaxation. Anesthetics (e.g. halothane) can inhibit the positive inotropic effect of calcium. Calcium has been used intraoperatively for its positive inotropic action, but its routine use, prophylactically, for protection against citrate intoxication, although still under consideration, has been generally abandoned.

There will be increasing numbers of patients, having received a calcium channel blocking drug (e.g. verapamil) for cardiac arrhythmias, in need of anesthetic management. The clinical implication is not well defined at present. However, it is reasonable to assume that such patients may have compromised myocardial performance through interference of calcium influx during depolarization. The combined use of verapamil and propranolol can have an additive effect on depression of AV conduction and myocardial contractility.

Magnesium

Magnesium is the second most abundant intracellular cation, having about 1/6 the concentration of potassium. The concentration in plasma is 1.5 to 2.2 mEq/L with about 2/3 as free cation and 1/3 bound to plasma protein. Magnesium is a co-factor for ATP in all its phosphate transfer reactions and is a co-factor for a large number of enzymes. However, it has not received the attention it deserves because the other cations are more conspicuously effected during anesthetic management.

The interaction of magnesium with other endogenous cations on electrophysiology is complex. Magnesium plays an important role in regulating calcium ion movement and distribution in cells, and is frequently overlooked during treatment of cardiac arrhythmias associated with hypokalemia and hypocalcemia. The neuromuscular depressant and vasodilation effects of exogenously administered $MgSO_4$ are better known to the anesthesiologist.

Hypomagnesemia can occur in diarrhea, chronic alcoholism, diabetes mellitus, renal tubular damage, diuretic therapy, and following hemodialysis or cardiopulmonary bypass. The clinical manifestations may include neuromuscular hyperactivity tremor and myoclonic jerks, convulsions and cardiac arrhythmias. The ECG changes associated with magnesium deficit are similar to those seen with hypercalcium. Magnesium deficiency may be associated with hypokalemia and enhanced toxicity to digitalis glycosides. Ventricular tachycardia refractory to potassium, procainamide, lidocaine, diphenylhydantoin and cardiac pacing but responded to $MgSO_4$. Failure to defibrillate in patients following cardiopulmonary bypass was successfully defibrillated with the administration of bolus doses of $MgSO_4$.

Hypermagnesemia is usually due to renal insufficiency, and is manifested by muscle weakness, hypotension, sedation and confusion. The toxemic patient, receiving $MgSO_4$, is another group of hypermagnesemic patients that the anesthesiologist must manage. Deep tendon reflexes are reduced when plasma [Mg^{++}] reaches 4 mEq/L and may be absent at levels approaching 10 mEq/L. At 12-15 mEq/L respiratory paralysis and AV conduction blocks are potential hazards. Intravenous $CaCl_2$ is the effective antagonist of magnesium overdose. The neurodepressant effect of Mg^{++} reduces the requirement for depolarizing as well as non-depolarizing neuromuscular blocking agents.

References

1. Aasheim GM: Hyponatremia during transurethral surgery. Canad Anaesth Soc J 20:274-280, 1973.
2. Antman EM, Stone PH, Mueller JE, et al: Calcium channel blocking agents in the treatment of cardiovascular disorders. Part I. Basic and clinical electrophysiologic effects. Annals of Internal Medicine 93:875-885, 1980.
3. Chadda KD, Lichstein E, Gupta P: Hypomagnesemia and refractory cardiac arrhythmias in non-digitalized patient. Am J Cardiol 31: 98-100, 1973.

4. Daniell HW: Arrhythmia in hypokalemia. N Engl J Med 284:1385, 1971.
5. Edmonds CJ, Jasani BM: Total body potassium changes with prolonged diuretic therapy. Am Heart J 85:569-571, 1973.
6. Ellrodt G, Chu CYC, Sing BN: Therapeutic implications of slow channel blockade in cardiocirculatory disorders. Circulation 62:669-679, 1980.
7. Ghoneim MM, Long JP: The interaction between magnesium and other neuromuscular blocking agents. Anesthesiology 32:23-27, 1970.
8. Giesecke AH, Morris RE, Dalton MD, et al: Of magnesium, muscle relaxants, toxemic parturients, and cats. Anesth Analg 47:689-695, 1968.
9. Gronert G, Theye RA: Pathophysiology of hyperkalemia induced by succinylcholine. Anesthesiology 43:89-99, 1975.
10. Hinkle JE, Cooperman LH: Serum ionized calcium changes following citrated blood transfusion in anesthetized man. Br J Anaesth 43: 1108-1112, 1971.
11. Jasani BM, Edmonds CJ: Kinetics of potassium distribution in man using isotope dilution and whole body counting. Metabolism 20:1099-1106, 1971.
12. Johnson JE, Hartsuch JM, Zollinger RM, et al: Radiopotassium equilibrium in total body potassium: Studies using ^{43}K and ^{42}K. Metabolism 18:663-668, 1969.
13. Kawamura R, Wong KC, Hodges MR: Intravenous potassium chloride in hypokalemic dogs pretreated with digoxin. Anesth Analg (Cleve) 57: 108-113, 1978.
14. Lawson NW, Butler GH, Rat CT: Alkalosis and cardiac arrhythmia. Anesth Analg (Cleve) 52:951-962, 1973.
15. Mazze RI, Escue HM, Houston JB: Hyperkalemia and cardiovascular collapse following administration of succinylcholine to traumatized patient. Anesthesiology 31:540-547, 1969.
16. Miller RD: Complications of massive blood transfusions. Anesthesiology 39:82-93, 1973.
17. Nayler WG: Calcium exchange in cardiac muscle: A basic mechanism of drug action. Am Heart J 73:379-394, 1967.
18. Price HL: Calcium reverses myocardial depression caused by halothane: Site of action. Anesthesiology 41:576-579, 1974.
19. Sack D, Kim ND, Harrison CE Jr: Contractility and subcellular calcium metabolism in chronic potassium deficiency. Am J Physiol 226:756-762, 1974.
20. Schernman MM, Sullivan RW, Hyatt KH: Magnesium metabolism in patients undergoing cardiopulmonary bypass. Circulation 39:(Suppl)235-241, 1969.
21. Scribner BH, Burnell JM: Interpretation of the serum potassium concentration. Metabolism 5:468-479, 1956.
22. Seller RH, Cangiano J, Kim KE, et al: Digitalis toxicity and hypomagnesemia. Am Heart J 79:57-68, 1970.
23. Tobey RE: Paraplegia, succinylcholine and cardiac arrest. Anesthesiology 32:359-364, 1970.
24. Tolmic JD, Joyce TH, Mitchess GD: Succinylcholine danger in the burned patient. Anesthesiology 28:467-470, 1967.
25. Viby-Mogensen J, Hanel HK, Hansen E, et al: Serum cholinesterase activity in burned patients. II. Anesthesia, suxamethonium and hyperkalaemia. Acta Anaesthesiol Scand 19:169-179, 1975.
26. Wills MR: The Biochemical Consequences of Chronic Renal Failure. Baltimore, University Park Press, 1971.
27. Wong KC, Kawamura R, Hodges MR, et al: Acute intravenous administration of potassium chloride to furosemide pretreated dogs. Canad Anaesth Soc J 24:203-211, 1977.

28. Wright BD, DiGiovanni AJ: Respiratory alkalosis, hypokalemia and repeated ventricular fibrillation associated with mechanical ventilation. Anesth Analg (Cleve) 48:467-473, 1969.

Reviews

1. Surawicz B, Gettes LS: Chapter 21: Effects of Electrolyte Abnormalities on the Heart and Circulation, pp 539-576. In Cardiac and Vascular Diseases edited by Conn HL Jr and Horwitz O. Lea & Febiger, 1971.
2. "Symposium on Body Fluid and Electrolyte Disorders" in Medical Clinics of North America, Vol 65, No 2, March 1981.

Table. Ionic Concentrations and Potentials in Mammalian Muscle Cells and Interstitial Fluid*

	Interstitial Fluid	Intracellular Fluid	$E = \frac{[ion]o}{[ion]i}$	$= \frac{60}{Z} \log \frac{[ion]o}{[ion]i}$ (mV)
Cations				
Na^+	145 um/cm^3	12 um/cm^3	12.1	65
K^+	4 um/cm^3	155 um/cm^3	1/39	-95
H^+	3.8×10^{-5} um/cm^3	13×10^{-5} um/cm^3	1/3.4	-32
[pH]	[7.43]	[6.9]		
Others	5 um/cm^3			
Anions				
Cl^-	120 um/cm^3	3.8 um/cm^3	31.8	-90
HCO_3	27 um/cm^3	8 um/cm^3	3.4	-32
Others	7 um/cm^3	155 um/cm^3		
Potential	0	-90 mV	31.6	-90

Adapted from Woodbury, 1962.

*o = extracellular; i = intracellular; Z = valence of ion.

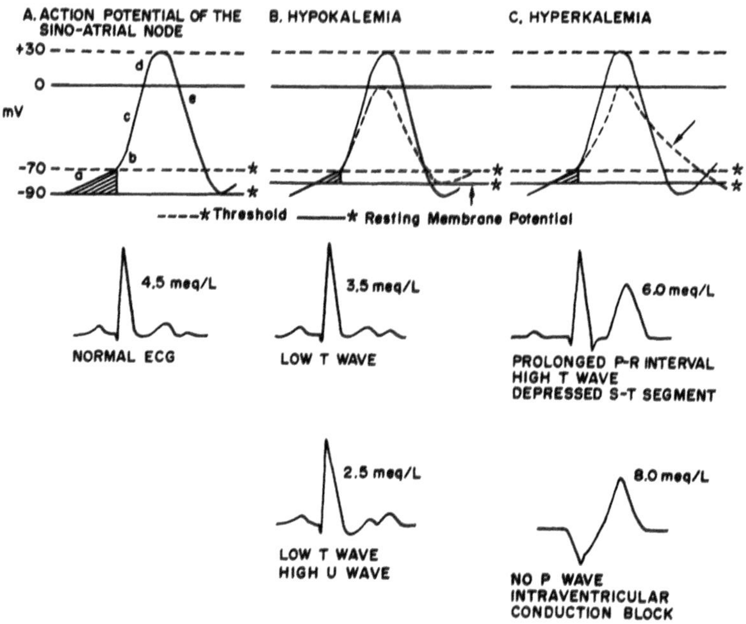

Figure. Serum potassium abnormality on the electrophysiology of the sinoatrial node and the ECG.

A. Action potential of normokalemic sinoatrial node
   a. Spontaneous depolarization (influx of Ca^{++} through slow channels)
   b. Threshold potential (open sodium gate)
   c. Maximal rate of depolarization (influx of Na^{+} through fast channels)
   d. Overshoot
   e. Repolarization (efflux of K^{+} through fast channels)

B. Action potential of chronic hypokalemic sinoatrial node. Intracellular potassium loss reduces (arrow) the resting membrane potential (more positive). A smaller action potential is produced. The shaded triangle area shows that less stimulus is required to excrete the cardiac cell.

C. Action potential of hyperkalemic sinoatrial node. Hyperkalemia reduces the resting membrane potential. As the hyperkalemia becomes more severe, depolarization as well as repolarization are inhibited.

Characteristic ECG changes with corresponding serum potassium changes are shown below the action potential.

ANESTHETIC MANAGEMENT OF THE HIGH RISK PREGNANT PATIENT: PREECLAMPSIA AND DIABETES

CHARLES P. GIBBS, M.D.

PREECLAMPSIA

Classification

Many classifications and terms have been used to define and identify the various hypertensive disorders of pregnancy. The following classification may be a useful one.

Hypertensive Disorders

I. Toxemia: A general non-specific, recently eschewed term used to describe all the various hypertensive disorders of pregnancy.

II. Preeclampsia (pregnancy-induced hypertension): A syndrome of hypertension, proteinuria and generalized edema occuring after the 20th week of gestation and usually abating within 48 hours of delivery.

A. Mild

1. Blood pressure: systolic blood pressure greater than 140, diastolic blood pressure greater than 90. A rise in systolic blood pressure of 30 mmHg or a rise in diastolic blood pressure of greater than 15 mmHg. These readings must be present on at least two separate occasions or at least 6 hours apart.
2. Proteinuria: greater than 0.3 g/liter on two random samples at least 6 hours apart.
3. Edema.

B. Severe

1. Blood pressure: 160/110 mmHg or greater.
2. Proteinuria greater than 5 grams per 24 hours.
3. Urine output less than 500 ccs per 24 hours and a rising creatinine level.
4. Pulmonary edema.
5. Persistent cerebral or visual disturbances.
6. Epigastric or right upper quadrant pain (indicating hepatic rupture).
7. Hepatocellular damage.
8. Severe thrombocytopenia or overt intravascular coagulation.

C. Eclampsia: preeclampsia with superimposed convulsions.

II. Chronic hypertension: the presence of persistent hypertension, regardless of etiology, before the 20th week of gestation or beyond 6 weeks postpartum.

III. Preeclampsia superimposed on chronic hypertension.

IV. Gestational hypertension: the development of hypertension without proteinuria or generalized edma during the last weeks of pregnancy or immediately postpartum.

V. Renal disease.

VI. Hypertension due to diseases of the adrenal madella or cortex.

Etiology

Multiple, multiple etiologies for preeclampsia-eclampsia have been proposed. None has been identified as the single cause. Preeclampsia is a disease characterized by generalized vasoconstriction. One current theory suggests that a poorly profused placenta, perhaps secondary to abnormal uterine artery structure, diminishes the capacity of the placenta to produce the vasodilatory prostaglandins A and E. Because of the lack of sufficient amounts of these prostaglandins, arteries are more susceptible to vasoconstrictive substances, particularly angiotensin II. Thus, hypertension and further reductions in uteroplacental blood flow occur. Tht sympathetic hyperactivity is not the eiology is made clear by the studies of Assali and Prystowksy who would not eliminate the hypertension with total sympathetic blockade provided by total spinal anesthesia.[1]

Whatever the etiology of preeclampsia, the manifestations of the disease are many, most of which are of great importance to the anesthesiologist. As the disease process worsens, these manifestations become more evident and more critical. Thus, for the the most part, this discussion will concentrate on the severe preeclamptic.

Manifestations

Features of the disease which are of importance to the anesthesiologist include the following.

I. The severe preeclamptic patient is a critically ill patient and must be considered as such. If this concept is accepted, then care and ultimate prognosis will be significantly improved.

II. Hypertension: Generalized vasospasm produces an increased peripheral vascular resistance resulting in hypertension.

III. Decreased uterine blood flow usually in proportion to severity of disease.[2,3]

IV. Decreased glomerular filtration rate.[4]

V. Hypovolemia: Secondary to the generalized vasoconstriction and is comparable to that seen in other hypertensive states. Pritchard and Stone have measured blood volume in normal pregnant and toxemic pregnant women and found the blood volume in the toxemia patients to be 27% lower.[5]

VI. Generalized and cerebral edema.[6]

VII. Decreased colloid osmotic pressure.[7]

VIII. Coagulopathies:[8]

A. Thrombocytopenia - 29%

B. Hypofibrogenemia - 8%

C. Prolonged plasma thrombin time - 50%

Obviously these changes must be taken into account when considering the use of regional anesthesia and/or central line placement.

IX. Treatment: Obstetric treatment may influence anesthetic management.

A. Bed rest.

B. Sedation.

C. Magnesium sulphate: This agent acts at the myoneural junction to inhibit the release of acetylcholine. It also produces a mild sedative effect and slight vasodilatation. It is used primarily to prevent convulsions and may be administered either intravenously or intramuscularly. Normal plasma levels are 1.5 to 2 meq/L. The therapeutic range is 4 to 6 meq/L. As an anticonvulsive agent it is very effective. As an antihypertensive it is very ineffective. Side effects include drowsiness, loss of deep tendon reflexes, EKG changes, respiratory paralysis and cardiac arrest. Respiratory paralysis should not occur until levels of 15 meq/L are reached. The antidote for magnesium-induced depression is calcium chloride or gluconate. Obviously, this agent is important to the anesthesiologist because it will enhance and prolong the effects of both succinylcholine and the non-depolarizing muscle relaxants.

D. Antihypertensives: The most common agents used by obstetricians are hydralazine and methyldopa.

X. Hypersensitivity to endogenous and exogenous vasopressor agents.[9,10,11]

IX. Causes of Death: The two most common causes of death are cerebral hemorrhage and pulmonary edema.[12]

Anesthetic Management

Mild preeclampsia: The mildly preeclamptic patient is a totally different person from the severely preeclamptic one. The cardiovascular changes are not nearly as marked. Thus, although caution must be taken, these patients will usually tolerate either regional or general anesthesia for cesarean section and would probably benefit from regional anesthesia during labor to make the laboring process as comfortable as possible. The risk of hypotension, provided the usual prophylactic measures are taken, is minimal.

Severe preeclampsia: Again, perhaps the most important aspect of dealing with these patients is to realize that many of them are critically ill. These patients will usually be treated with bed rest, sedation and magnesium sulphate as preliminary, conservative measures by the obstetricians. If, after a brief trial of these measures, the patient does not improve, antihypertensive medication, usually in the form of hydralazine will be initiated. The aim of most therapy is to prevent convulsions and to maintain diastolic blood pressure below 100 mmHg.

The contribution of the anesthesiologist to these patients is twofold: Help evaluate and optimize overall condition of the patient and provide pain relief.

1. Evaluating and optimizing overall condition of the patient in as short a time as possible is of primary importance. Only when proper preparation and stabilization has occurred can appropriate decisions about pain relief be made. Proper evaluation and preparation will include the following:
   a. Volume status: To determine the volume status either a Swan-Ganz catheter or a CVP line must be placed. Many of these patients will be found to have CVP measurements of 1-2 centimeters of water.[13,14] Before any regional technique is instituted the volume status must

be normalized. In some instances 1-2 liters of crystalloid solution will bring CVP measurements to 6-8 centimeters of water. In others, crystalloids will not be enough, and either albumin or plasmanate will be necessary because crystalloid does not stay in the intravascular space except for a brief time even in normal patients.[15] In these patients with decreased oncotic pressure and perhaps leaky vessels, it is even more likely that the crystalloid will diffuse out of the intravascular space, thus creating the need for colloid solutions. Several recent reports in the literature have emphasized the superiority of colloid solutions over crystalloid as a means for maintaining intravascular volume.[13,15,16] Usually, with the re-establishment of a normal blood volume, urine output will increase, and blood pressure will decrease toward normal.[13,16] For the more complicated patient, several authors have found the Swan-Ganz catheter to be more accurate and useful.[17-22]

b. Blood pressure monitoring: An arterial line is necessary to monitor the status of the blood pressure under either regional or general anesthesia. These patients are subject to wide swings of blood pressure and these wide swings need to be treated promptly and effectively.[22]

c. Urine output: A Foley catheter should be inserted so that an accurate account can be kept of this important vital sign.

d. Clotting profile: If the clotting profile is abnormal, regional anesthesia is contraindicated. Thus, small incremental doses of narcotics will need to be used for labor and inhalational analgesia plus a pudendal block must suffice for vaginal delivery. General anesthesia is indicated for cesarean section.

The above represent the most important steps in the adequate preparation of the preeclamptic patient. Obviously, there are many other bits of information that need be known and are usually gathered by the obstetrician, for example, electrolytes, BUN, hematocrit, etc.

Lumbar epidural for labor and vaginal delivery: The following represents a series of steps that may be used as guidelines for providing regional anesthesia for the severely preeclamptic patient during labor and vaginal delivery.

1. Check coagulation profile.
2. Optimize volume status and blood pressure as described above. (CVP should be at 6-8 centimeters of water or pulmonary wedge pressure should be at 8-12 millimeters of mercury).
3. Electronic fetal monitoring: Regional anesthesia should not be carried out in these patients without being aware of fetal status at all times.
4. Lateral recumbent or sitting position.
5. Atraumatic epidural tap at L3-4 or L4-5. Thread catheter no more than 2-4 centimeters.
6. Test dose with 3 ccs of 1.5% lidocaine, 3% chloroprocaine, or 0.75% bupivacaine with 1:200,000 epinephrine.[23] (May want to avoid because of a rise in blood pressure with epinephrine.)
7. Loading dose: 3-5 ccs of 1% lidocaine, 2% 2-chloroprocaine or .25% bupivacaine. The aim here is to establish a segmental epidural block, i.e., a block that produces a band of analgesia at the T10-L1-2 level.
8. Top up doses with 1/2 original dose by the clock to minimize tachyphylaxis.
9. Maintain left lateral position throughout labor. Right lateral position may be acceptable, but

supine position should be avoided. For vaginal delivery:

1. Elevate head of bed or place patient in sitting position and inject 6-10 ccs of 1.5% lidocaine or 3% chloroprocaine.

Lumbar epidural for cesarean section:

1. Optimization and stabilization is the same as above.
2. A clear antacid such as sodium citrate or Bicitra should be given in event general anesthesia is necessary.[24,25,26]
3. Test dose as above.
4. Loading dose: 15-20 ccs of 1.5% lidocaine, 3% chloroprocaine or 0.5% bupivicaine. These loading doses should be given as incremental doses of 5-6 ccs at a time.[20]
5. Maintain left uterine displacement. Treat falling blood pressure immediately.[21] Do not wait for "hypotension" to develop. As soon as the systolic blood pressure drops 10 mmHg, fluids should be increased. If this simple measure is not effective, small doses of ephedrine may be given. Initial doses of ephedrine should not exceed five milligrams because these patients are hypersensitive to vasopressor agents.[7,8]

General anesthesia for cesarean section:

1. Again optimization and stabilization as for regional anesthesia.

2. Preoperative antacids: 0.3 M sodium citrate or Bicitra 30 ccs.[24,25,26]

3. Prevent cardiovascular effects of laryngoscopy and intubation by administering an intravenous antihypertensive agent. Because these patients may become quite agitated on arrival to the operating room, these antihypertensive agents may need to be started as preparation for the operation

begins. Usually however, it will suffice to begin a slow infusion at the time of preoxygenation. The slow infusion is maintained until a short time after intubation is accomplished. Blood pressure is not necessarily lowered but maintained at a level not exceeding those which existed before being brought to the operating room.

a. Nitroprusside: This agent is quite effective. However, it has produced cyanide toxicity in fetal lambs when administered to the maternal ewe.[27] The toxicity occurred in fetuses of ewes who had demonstrated tachyphylaxis to the drug. Others have more recently reported favorable results following nitroprusside administration to pregnant ewes.[28] Cyanide levels remained below 50 ug/ml in both mothers fetuses. Because the amount used is so small, and the duration of its use is so short, it is unlikely that such toxicity would occur in the human infant. We and others have used this agent on multiple occasions and found it to be both effective and safe.[29]

b. Trimethaphan: This agent is another short acting antihypertensive agent which enjoys some popularity. Because it is a highly charged molecule it will not cross the placenta easily. However, because it is at least partially destroyed by cholinesterases, it will potentiate the action of succinylcholine.

c. Nitroglycerin: Although this agent is relatively free of complications, its effectiveness in the acute situation where blood pressures need to be lowered rapidly is not as good as the above two agents.

4. Preoxygenation.
5. Precurarization.
6. Thiopental 3-4 milligrams per kilogram.
7. Cricoid pressure.

8. Succinylcholine.
9. Laryngoscopy and intubation.
10. Check breath sounds.
11. Nitrous oxide 50/50 with oxygen.
12. 0.5% halothane.
13. Succinylcholine drip.
14. Oxytocin: 10-40 units in a liter. Avoid ergot drugs because of hypersensitivity to vasopressors.
15. Narcotic supplement following delivery of the infant.
16. Awake extubation: This process may also require the use of short acting intravenous and hypertensive agents.
17. To recovery room.

Recovery

The last item "to recovery room" needs discussion. Ideally the patient should be taken to a place where personnel and facilities are adequate to manage a severely ill person. Usually, this would require an intensive care unit setting where personnel are familiar with the extensive monitoring required. However, some hospitals may have such conditions available in either the recovery room or on the labor and delivery floor itself.

Postpartum

Following delivery many of these patients will have a decreased urine output, and it is here where proper monitoring of volume status is most helpful. Without adequate knowledge of the central blood volume, the patient may be presumed to be in renal shutdown when in reality she may be severely volume depleted. Such a differentiation is most important to insure proper treatment.

Summary

The severely preeclamptic patient represents an enigma and a challenge. Although the etiology of preeclampsia may not be forthcoming for some time, management can be considerably enhanced if we continue to remember that the patient is severely and critically ill and must be treated as such.

DIABETES

Diabetes is a metabolic disorder characterized primarily by hyperglycemia plus alterations in protein and lipid metabolism. It rates as the most common medical complication of pregnancy, occurring once in every 700 to 1000 gestations.[1,2] Eighty to ninety percent of these patients manifest gestational diabetes, a carbohydrate intolerance which appears for the first time during pregnancy and resolves after delivery, while 10 percent have a prior history of insulin dependence.[3]

Ketoacidosis and postpartum hypoglycemia represent the major maternal threats to the pregnant diabetic woman.[4] Ketoacidosis is associated with a maternal mortality rate of 5 to 15 percent and a perinatal mortality rate of 30 to 70 percent. Ketoacidosis occurs most often late in pregnancy when insulin demands are greatest, while hypoglycemia occurs postpartum when insulin demands fall suddenly and drastically. The higher incidence of pregnancy induced hypertension, 25 to 30 percent, also contributes to maternal mortality and morbidity.[5]

A 75 percent reduction in perinatal mortality has been observed in pregnancies complicated by diabetes during the past 10 years.[6-8] The current overall perinatal mortality rate for the insulin dependent patient is approximately 5 to 6 percent.[9-11] Even more encouraging is the fact that many centers have reported perinatal mortality rates no higher in the insulin dependent diabetic than in normal gestations. This improved outcome has been due to advances in neonatal care, better techniques for antepartum fetal surveillance and assessment of fetal maturation, and attention to meticulous control of maternal diabetes. However, congenital malformations, the leading cause of perinatal mortality today, remain an unsolved problem.

<u>Pathophysiology of diabetes:</u>

A. Glucose is needed by cells for energy source and is absorbed from gut into the blood stream and taken to the liver which:
   1. Releases it for utilization by tissues.
   2. <u>or</u> stores it as glycogen (short term).
   3. <u>or</u> if excessive glucose is present converts it to fat which is stored in fat cells.

B. Insulin
   1. Enhances transfer of glucose across cell membranes (except in brain) and thus:
      a. Increases glucose metabolism.
      b. Decreases blood glucose concentration.
      c. Increases glycogen synthesis (mostly in liver).

C. Hyperglycemia, the cardinal feature of diabetes, occurs for two reasons:
   1. Overproduction of glucose by liver via:
      a. Dietary CHO.
      b. Liver Glycogen.
      c. Gluconeogenesis from amino acids and glycerol.
   2. Peripheral underutilization of glucose secondary to decreased circulating insulin. Peripheral underutilization cause the following sequence of events:
      a. Underutilization by muscle - loss of muscle glycogen and release of amino acids for gluconeogenesis.
      b. Underutilization by adipose tissue leads to:
         1. Impaired triglyceride metabolism.
         2. Release of free fatty acids into blood stream - part of which are converted to ketone bodies by liver.
      c. Ketone bodies build up in blood as does glucose and overflow into urine.

d. Body loses glucose, ketone bodies, water, and base.

e. Thus, dehydration, ketoacidosis, weight loss, coma and death may ensue.

Effects of Pregnancy on Diabetes

Pregnacy alters carbohydrate metabolism in two ways. First, pregancy promotes a state of accelerated starvation during which blood levels of glucose and amino acids decrease while free fatty acids and ketone bodies increase. In addition, the insulin response to a given glucose load is increased. This state of accelerated starvation is probably explained by the utilization of glucose by the fetus. Glucose is the most important fetal fuel and traverses the placenta from the mother promoting hypoglycemia. Amino acids also reach the fetus and may be utilized for protein synthesis.

The second way in which pregnancy alters carbohydrate metabolism is by creating a diabetogenic state. While the previously described accelerated starvation state is more evident during the earlier parts of pregnancy, the diabetogenic stress is more important during the latter half of pregnancy. This diabetogenic state is manifested by:

1. A decreased response to exogenous insulin.
2. An increase in postprandial blood sugars.
3. The onset of gestational diabetes in women with inadequate pancreatic reserve.

Such a disturbed metabolic pattern results because the placenta produces anti-insulin enzymes as well as human placental lactogen (HPL).[12,13,14,15] This hormone resembles growth hormone in structure and increases maternal lipolysis resulting in maternal utilization of fat for energy with sparing of glucose for fetal consumption. The placenta also produces increasing amounts of estrogen and progesterone which alter maternal islet cell function which produces beta-cell hyperplasia and maternal hyperinsulinemia.[16-18] Importantly, because these effects are mediated via the placenta, they disappear shortly after birth.

Because the anti-insulin factors are at work during pregnancy, the maternal organism responds by producing more insulin for a given glucose load. A normal pregnant patient will be able to respond to this added stress. However, a person who is a borderline or covert diabetic may not be able to do so. Thus, pregnancy provides the stress that will unmask this "prediabetic" state which is referred to as gestational diabetes.

Also as a result of the anti-insulin factors, the insulin-dependent patient will require increases in insulin dosages during pregnancy, particularly during the latter half when the insulin antagonists are at their highest levels.[19] During this time the insulin needs may increase by 70%.[20]

Another feature of pregnancy which needs emphasis is that insulin does not cross the placenta. Therefore, although the fetus receives a continuous supply of maternal glucose, maternal insulin will not accompany the glucose. During the diabetic pregnancy, the hypoinsulinemic mother becomes hyperglycemic. The excess glucose will cross to the fetus leading to stimulation of the fetal pancreatic beta cells which will result in beta cell hyperplasia and subsequently fetal hyperinsulinemia. Thus, the fetus is subjected to both hyperglycemia and hyperinsulinemia, factors which lead to much of the morbidity and mortality seen in the infant of the diabetic mother (IDM). The combination of excess glucose and insulin will produce fetal macrosomia.[21] Intrauterine deaths characteristic of the diabetic pregnancy may be linked to the hyperglycemia and hyperinsulinemia as well.[22] Moreover, this combination may alter fetal lung development in surfactant synthesis which increases the likelihood of the respiratory distress syndrome.[23]

Pregnancy Outcome: Perhaps the most widely used system for assessing the outcome or predicting the outcome of diabetic pregnancies is that devised by White.[1] The system or classification is based on factors known prior to pregnancy including the age of onset of diabetes, its duration, the use of insulin and the presence or absence of vascular disease. Her classification is as follows:

Class	Age of onset (yr)		Duration (yr)	Vascular disease	Insulin
A	Any		Pregnancy	0	0
B	>20		<10	0	+
C	10-19	or	10-19	0	+
D	<10	or	>20	Benign retinopathy	+
F	Any		Any	Nephropathy	+
R	Any		Any	Proliferative retinopathy	+
H	Any		Any	Heart Disease	+

In addition to the White classification Pedersen has developed a set of characteristics called the Prognostically Bad Signs of Pregnancy or PBSP.[6,7] These signs include clinical findings such as phelonephritis, ketoacidosis, pregnancy induced hypertension, and neglect or failure to follow a recommended therapeutic regimen. The combination of White's and Pedersen's criteria provides particularly useful predictive data.

Laboratory diagnosis of diabetes: The values used for diagnosing diabetes during pregnancy are somewhat different than those used in the nonpregnant state. Upper limit values most widely used during pregnancy are as follows:

	Whole blood[24] (mg/dl)	Plasma[25] (mg/dl)
Screening test		
50 gm, 1 hr.	130	140
Oral GTT		
Fasting	90	105
1 hr.	165	190
2 hr.	145	165
3 hr.	125	145

Clinical management of the insulin dependent patient: Control of maternal glucose levels within normal physiologic limits is the most important therapeutic goal. During normal pregnancy maternal glucose levels rarely exceed 100 mg/dl except for brief periods after meals. Fasting levels usually range from 60 to 80 mg/dl.[26] Control of maternal glycemia within this range has produced low perinatal mortality rates and perinatal morbidity. For example, Karlson and Kjellmer achieved a perinatal mortality rate of 38 per 1000 when maternal glucose levels were kept below 100 mg/dl.[27] However, when mean glucose levels exceeded 100 mg/dl mortality rose six-fold. Monitoring of blood glucose is usually done on a daily basis using a glucose reflectance meter and glucose oxidase impregnated strips.[28,29,30] Monitoring urinary glucose excretion often proves inadequate in pregnancies since renal glycosuria, a consequence of a normally increased glomerular filtration rate, occurs frequently during pregnancy. Recently, levels of hemoglobin A, a hemoglobin whose level reflects chronic hyperglycemia, has been used to provide a retrospective appraisal of the severity of the diabetic state.[31]

Timing of the delivery of the insulin-dependent diabetic is critical. Because of the increased risk of fetal and/or perinatal morbidity, diabetic pregnancies are not allowed beyond term. Nevertheless, the obstetrician must be certain that the fetus has reached sufficient maturity to preclude the development of RDS. Multiple tests and evaluations are necessary throughout pregnancy and become even more critical as term approaches. Because many of these patients will have their labors induced, and because some inductions will fail as well as initiate fetal distress, the cesarean section rate is high in these patients. Currently, approximately 50% of all insulin-dependent patients undergo cesarean section.[9,10]

Management during labor and delivery: During labor and delivery, maternal glucose levels must be carefully regulated to prevent subsequent neonatal hypoglycemia. Maternal hyperglycemia will produce neonatal hyperglycemia and then hyperinsulinemia which persists after the glucose is gone - leading to neontal hypoglycemia. Lucas has recently reported that normal women who received 10 to 20 g. of glucose per hour for over 4 hours delivered infants with significantly higher plasma insulin concentrations.[32] Furthermore, Light and coworkers have demonstrated a significantly greater incidence of neonatal hypoglycemia in IDMs whose blood sugars exceeded 140 mg/ml.[33] To maintain lower blood sugar levels, an intravenous infusion of 5 percent dextrose solution should run at rates no greater than 150 ml/hr. On the day of induction or cesarean section, several insulin regimens may be utilized.[1,34] The patient may receive one-half to one-third of her usual pre-pregnancy insulin dose in the form of long acting or NPH insulin. After delivery, the patient's insulin requirement falls markedly and maternal hypoglycemia can result. At the present time, many clincians prefer continuous intravenous infusion of insulin and glucose during the induction of labor.[35,36] Ten units of regular insulin may be added to a 1000 ml infusion bottle of 5 percent glucose and given to the patient at a rate of approximately 100 ml/hr. At the start of the infusion, maternal glucose levels should be assessed hourly and followed at 3 to 4 hour intervals once the patient becomes stable. This monitoring may be carried out most easily using a glucose reflectance meter. Insulin is usually withheld if an elective cesarean section is scheduled. Blood glucose is monitored closely after delivery and short acting insulin given as needed.

Insulin types

Action	Insulin	Duration of action, hr	Peak effect, hr postinjection
Fast	Crystalline zinc= clear=(regular)= soluble	6	2-3
	Semilente	12	3-6
Inter-	Globin	18	6-8
mediate	NPH	24	8-12
	Lente	24	8-12
Long	Ultralente	36	20-30
	Protamine zinc	36	16-24

Management of severe ketoacidosis: Ketoacidosis presents two major problems: metabolic acidosis and dehydration. Metabolic acidosis results from the accumulation of beta-hydroxybutyric acid and acetic acid in the bloodstream which produces a fall in pH and serum bicarbonate. Glucose accumulates concomitantly with the development of metabolic acidosis. Both the metabolic acidosis and the accumulation of glucose result from the underutilization of insulin. The marked hyperglycemia that ensues causes an osmotic diuresis with its attendant loss of water and electrolytes leading to dehydration. A suspected diagnosis of ketoacidosis calls for a complete blood count and determination of blood glucose, urea nitrogen, electrolytes, and serum ketones. An arterial blood gas is obtained for measurement of pH, carbon dioxide, and oxygen tensions. Treatment aims at correcting the basic abnormality in metabolism by providing adequate insulin, restoration of water and electrolyte losses, and identification of precipitating factors. A separate, precise record of the various treatments and responses helps to assess the degree of progress quickly and coherently. Regular insulin can be administered in relatively large doses of 100 units initially, followed by doses of 50 to 100 units every 2 to 4 hours until blood glucose levels fall to 250 mg/100 ml. Usually half the original dose is given intravenously. Blood sugar levels, electrolytes, arterial pH, and blood gas tensions are repeated at least every 2 hours. Recently, much smaller doses of insulin have been effective when administered as a continuous infusion.[37] Linzey has utilized a regimen of 10 units of regular insulin given intravenously, followed by a constant infusion of 6 units of insulin per hour.[35] Early reports suggested the need for an infusion pump and the addition of human albumin to prevent adherence of insulin to the tubing. However, recent data suggest equal effectiveness when eliminating the albumin and employing a pediatric infusion set.[36,37] The infusion of 1.5 liters of normal saline during the first 60 minutes followed by 500 to 1000 ml per hour corrects dehydration.[38] If necessary, central venous pressure monitoring is used. Since the correction of the metabolic abnormality by the appropriate administration of insulin will prevent the formation of additional acid byproducts and, therefore, the development of further acidosis, the use of bicarbonate is not indicated unless the acidosis is severe. Severe acidosis necessitates treatment with bicarbonate to prevent the deleterious effects of acidemia on myocardial contractility. When bicarbonate is administered, it is given in a dose calculated as one-half the base deficit. Felig has recommended that the acidosis need not be treated until the pH falls below 7.1.[39] Because sodium bicarbonate has a very high osmolarity, it is given as an infusion in 0.45 percent saline to prevent further celular dehydration. Acidosis, diuresis, and frequent vomiting cause a loss of potassium. Blood levels may not reflect the potassium loss because acidosis will draw potassium from the cells, thus creating a deceptively high blood level. Following the correction of acidosis, potassium will re-enter the cells and hypokalemia will become evident. Therefore, potassium need may not become obvious until 3 to 4 hours after initiation of treatment. When necessary, potassium chloride can be administered in a dose of 40 mEq/liter of intravenous fluid. A total of 120 to 160 mEq can be infused in the first 12 to 18 hours.[39] Both the electrocardiogram and serum potassium levels are helpful in estimating the potassium deficit and in following potassium therapy.

Anesthetic management for labor and vaginal delivery is not complicated if the physician observes the above features of the disease. Small doses of intravenous narcotics or a methoxyflurane inhaler will provide moderate and safe analgesia for patients without renal damage. Lumbar epidural analgesia for labor and delivery or spinal analgesia for delivery will safely provide excellent pain relief if maximal efforts are utilized to avoid the low incidence of hypotension that accompanies these techniques. During regional analgesia, a separate intravenous line for the administration of nondextrose containing fluids is necessary to prevent hypotension and still avoid hyperglycemia. Severe diabetics require particular attention because the IDM seems particularly susceptible to hypotension, a consideration to be discussed below.[40,41] Insulin management has been discussed previously for labor and delivery.

Anesthetic management for cesarean section: Anesthesia for cesarean section in the pregnant diabetic patient requires further consideration. The patient should be first on the operating schedule and blood sugar and electrolyte determinations obtained shortly before operation. As above, insulin is usually withheld prior to an elective cesarean section. In some institutions, the parturient receives one-half of her usual daily dose of long acting insulin early in the morning of the scheduled cesarean section. In either instance, blood glucose levels are measured frequently, using a glucose reflectance meter. Withholding all insulin in the morning and administering small doses of regular insulin during the procedure has the advantage of avoiding difficulties immediately postpartum when insulin requirements decline rapidly. Intravenous short acting insulin has a half-life of 3 to 3.5 min and thus affords the physician greater control.[42] Again, two intravenous lines will be necessary, one for glucose infusion and another for fluids and drugs. As during labor and vaginal delivery, the glucose solution should run at a rate no greater than 150 mg/hr. The intravenous preloading solution used to prevent hypotension should not contain glucose. Kenepp and colleagues have recently demonstrated that the administration of 1000 ml of dextrose-containing solutions as a preload infusion in normal mothers undergoing cesarean section will raise maternal glucose to 245 mg/dl. In a comparable group of patients receiving 1000 ml of normal saline, the maternal glucose remained at the preinfusion level, 75 mg/dl. In that study, the newborns of the mothers who had received the glucose solution had an averge blood sugar at 22 hours of 35 mg/dl compared with a mean blood sugar of 65 mg/dl in the group receiving normal saline.[43] During the procedure and immediately afterward, regular insulin is administered as needed in small doses. Ten units of intravenous regular insulin will lower the blood sugar approximately 75 to 100 mg/dl.

Until recently, little information existed regarding the choice of regional or general anesthesia for cesarean section in diabetic patients. Datta and coworkers have compared regional and general anesthesia in four groups of patients: (1) healthy patients receiving general anesthesia;(2) healthy patients receiving spinal analgesia; (3) diabetics receiving general anestheisa; and (4) diabetics receiving spinal analgesia. They found that infants of diabetic mothers receiving spinal analgesia did less well than infants of diabetic mothers receiving general anesthesia and less well than both groups of infants of healthy mothers.[40] Close inspection of the results revealed that the IDMs whose mothers had experienced hypotension during regional analgesia were the most severely affected. Since infants of normal mothers who had experienced comparable degrees of hypotension were not adversely affected, this work indicates that the IDM may be particularly sensitive to the harmful effects of hypotension. Another more recent study by the same authors evaluated epidural analgesia and, although the format of the study differed somewhat, the findings were similar.[41] In still another and even more recent study these same authors now provide data indicating that regional anesthesia can be used with no adverse effects on the fetus in the diabetic patient provided no hypotension occurs.[44] In this last study the authors not only used the customary methods of preventing hypotension, but they also treated a slightly falling systolic blood pressure. That is, they administered ephedrine to any patient whose systolic blood pressure decreased by 10 mmHg, thus preventing what is commonly referred to as hypotension. These three studies will not surprise those who believe that the fetus of the severe diabetic woman is a fetus in distress whose compensatory reserves may be severely depleted and who may not be able to cope with the additional insult of hypotension. Another method of preventing hypotension with reasonable certainty appears to be the addition of 5% albumin to the loading intravenous solution.[45] Finally, if hypotension can be reliably prevented or avoided, then regional anesthesia can be safely used in the pregnant diabetic patient.

General anesthesia, in the form of a balanced technique is also appropriate providing the peculiarities of the diabetic state are noted and appropriate measures taken to deal with them as described above.

REFERENCES - PREECLAMPSIA

1. Assali NS, Prystowsky H: Studies on autonomic blockade. II. Observations on the nature of blood pressure fall with high selective spinal anesthesia in pregnant women. J Clin Invest 29:1367, 1950.

2. Dixon HG, Browne JCM, Davey DA: Choriodecidual and myometrial blood-flow. Lancet 2:369, 1963.
3. Johnson T, Clayton CG: Diffusion of radioactive sodium in normotensive and pre-eclamptic pregnancies. Br Med J 1:312, 1957.
4. Chesley LC: Hypertensive Disorders in Pregnancy. New York, Appleton-Century-Crofts, 1978, pp 445-476.
5. Pritchard JA, Stone SR: Clinical and laboratory observations on eclampsia. Am J Obstet Gynecol 99:754, 1967.
6. Benedetti TJ, Quilligan EJ: Cerebral edema in severe pregnancy-induced hypertension. Am J Obstet Gynecol 137:860, 1980.
7. Benedetta TJ, Carlson RW: Studies of colloid osmotic pressure in pregnancy-induced hypertension. Am J Obstet Gynecol 135:308, 1979.
8. Pritchard JA, Cunningham FG, Mason RA: Coagulation changes in eclampsia: Their frequency and pathogenesis. Am J Obstet Gynecol 124:855, 1976.
9. Zuspan FP, Nelson GH, Ahlquist RP: Epinephrine infusions in normal and toxemic pregnancy. Am J Obstet Gynecol 90:88, 1964.
10. Gant NF, Daley GL, Chand S, et al: A study of angiotension II pressor response throughout primigravid pregnancy. J Clin Invest 52:2682, 1973.
11. Dieckmann WJ, Michel HL: Vascular-renal effects of posterior pituitary extracts in pregnant women. Am J Obstet Gynecol 33:131, 1937.
12. Covan ADT: The pathogenesis of eclamptic lesions. Patholigia et Microbiologia 24:562, 1961 (Supple.).
13. Joyce TH, Debnath KS, Baker EA: Preeclampsia - relationship of CVP and epidural analgesia. Anesthesiology 51 (3S):S297, 1979.
14. Cloeren SE, Lippert TH, Hinselmann M: Hypovolemia in toxemia of pregnancy: Plasma expander therapy with surveillance of central venous pressure. Arch Gynak, 215:123, 1973.
15. Shoemaker WC: Crystalloids, colloids, and blood products. ASA Refresher Course, pp 126B, 1981.
16. Sehgal NN, Hitt JR: Plasma volume expansion in the treatment of pre-eclampsia.
17. Paust JC, Reddy MAK: Swan-Ganz catheterization - an aid in management of high risk obstetrical patients. J of Kentucky Med Assoc 76:319, 1978.
18. Benedetti TJ, Cotton DB, Read JC, et al: Hemodynamic observations in severe pre-eclampsia with flow-directed pulmonary artery catheter. Am J Obstet Gynecol 136:465, 1980.
19. Hodgkinson R, Husain FJ, Hayashi RH: Systemic and pulmonary blood pressure during cesarean section in
20. Strauss RG, Keefer JR, Burke T, et al: Hemodynamic monitoring of cardiogenic pulmonary edema complicating toxemia of pregnancy. Obstet Gynecol 55:170, 1980.

21. Rafferty TD, Berkowitz RL: Hemodynamics in patients with severe toxemia during labor and delivery. Am J Obstet Gynecol 138:263, 1980.
22. Freund U, French W, Carlson RW, et al: Hemodynamic and metabolic studies of a case of toxemia of pregnancy. Am J Obstet Gynecol 127:206, 1977.
23. Moore DC, Batra MS: The components of an effective testdose prior to epidural block. Anesthesiology 55:696, 1981.
24. Gibbs CP, Hemling RE, Wynne JW, et al: Antacid pulmonary aspiration. Anesthesiology 51:S290, 1979.
25. Gibbs CP, Spohr L, Schmidt D: The effectiveness of sodium citrate as an antacid. Anesthesiology 57:44, 1982.
26. Eyler SW, Cullen BF, Murphy ME, et al: Antacid aspiration in rabbits: A comparison of mylanta and bicitra. Anesth Analg 61:288, 1982.
27. Naulty J, Cefalo RC, Lewis PE: Fetal toxicity of nitroprusside in the pregnant ewe. Am J Obstet Gynecol 139:78, 1981.
28. Ellis SC, Wheeler AS, James FM, III: Fetal and maternal effects of sodium nitroprusside used to counteract hypertension in gravid ewes. Am J Obstet Gynecol 143:766, 1982.
29. Stempel JE, O'Grady JP, Morton MJ, et al: Use of sodium nitroprusside in complications of gestational hypertension. Obstet Gynecol 60:533, 1982. parturients with gestational hypertension. Can Anaesth Soc J 27:389, 1980.

REFERENCES - DIABETES

1. White P: Pregnancy and diabetes: Medical aspects. Med Clin N Am 49:1015, 1965.
2. Felig P: Diabetes mellitus, in Burrow, GN and Ferris TF (eds.): Medical Complications during Pregnancy W.B. Sauders Co., Philadelphia, 1975.
3. Report of the Work Group on Pregnancy of the Committee on Scope and Impact to the National Committee on Diabetes, 1975, pp 180-181.
4. Gabbe SG, Mestman JH, Hibbard LT: Maternal mortality in diabetes mellitus. Obstet Gynecol 48:549, 1976.
5. Pedersen J: The Pregnant Diabetic and Her Newborn, 2nd ed. Williams and Wilkins, Balitmore, 1977.
6. Pedersen J, Molsted-Pedersen L, Andersen B: Assessors of fetal perinatal mortality in diabetic pregnancy. Diabetes 23:302, 1974.
7. White P: Classification of obstetric diabetes. Am J Obstet Gynecol 130:228, 1978.

8. Gyves MT, et al: A modern approach to management of pregnant diabetics: A two-year analysis of perinatal outcomes. Am J Obstet Gynecol 128:606, 1977.
9. Kitzmiller JL, et al: Diabetic pregnancy and perinatal morbidity. Am J Obstet Gynecol 131:560, 1978.
10. Gabbe SG, et al: Management and outcome of pregnancy in diabetes mellitus, classes B to R. Am J Obstet Gynecol 129:723, 1977.
11. Gugliucci CL, et al: Intensive care of the pregnant diabetic. Am J Obstet Gynecol 125:435, 1976.
12. Freinkel N, Goodner CJ: Carbohydrate metabolism in pregnancy. I. The metabolism of insulin by human placental tissue. J Clin Invest 39:116, 1960.
13. Posner, BI: Insulin metabolizing enzyme activities in human placental tissue. Diabetes 22:552, 1973.
14. Beck P, Daughaday WH: Human placental lactogen. Studies of its acute metabolic effects and disposition in normal man. J. Clin Invest 46:103, 1967.
15. Spellacy WN, Cohn JE: Human placental lactogen levels and daily insulin requirements in patients with diabetes mellitus complicating pregnancy. Obstet Gynecol 42:330, 1973.
16. Kalkhoff RK, Kissebah AH, Kim HJ: Carbohydrate and lipid metabolism during normal pregnancy: Relationship to gestational hormone action. Semin. Perinatol 2:291, 1978.
17. Frantz AG, Rabkin MT: Effects of estrogen and sex difference on secretion of human growth hormone. J Clin Endocrinol Metab 25:1470, 1965.
18. Beck P, Hoff DL: Oestriol modification and the effects of progesterone and human chorionic somatomammotrophin on glucose tolerance and plasma insulin in rhesus monkeys. Diabetes 20:271, 1971.
19. Spellacy WN, Goetz FC: Plasma insulin in normal late pregnancy. N Eng J Med 268:988, 1963.
20. Tyson JE, Felig P: Medical aspects of diabetes in pregnancy and the diabetogenic effectc of oral contraceptives. Med Clin N Am 55:947, 1971.
21. Whitelaw A: Subcutaneous fat in newborn infants of diabetec mothers: An indication of quality of diabetes control. Lancet 1:15, 1977.
22. Shelley HJ, Bassett JM, Milner RDG: Control of carbohydrate metabolism in the fetus and newborn. Br Med Bull 31:39, 1975.
23. Smith BT, et al: Insulin antagonism of cortisol action on lecithin synthesis by cultured fetal lung cells. J Pediatr 87:953, 1975.
24. O'Sullivan JB, et al: Screening criteria for high-risk gestational diabetic patients. Am J Obstet Gynecol 116:895, 1973.
25. Mastman J: Medical management of the pregnant diabetic. Contemp Obstet Gynecol 1:61, 1973.
26. Gillmer MDG, et al: Carbohydrate metabolism in pregnancy. I. Diurnal plasma glucose profile in normal and diabetic women. Br Med J 3:399, 1975.

27. Karlsson K, Kjellmer I: The outcome of diabetic pregnancies in relation to the mother's blood sugar level. Am J Obstet Gynecol 112:213, 1972.
28. Howe-Davies, S, et al: Home blood sampling for plasma glucose assay in control of diabetes. Br Med J 2:596, 1978.
29. Jovanovic L, et al: Feasibility of maintaining normal glucose profiles in insulin-dependent pregnant diabetic women. Am J Med68:105, 1980.
30. Schneider JM et al: Pregnancy complicating ambulatory patient management of diabetes. Diabetes Care 3:77, 1980.
31. Schwartz HC, et al: Effects of pregnancy on hemoglobin A_{1c} in normal, gestational diabetic and diabetic women. Diabetes 25:1118, 1976.
32. Lucas A, et al: Iatrogenic hyperinsulinism at birth. Lancet 1:44, 1980.
33. Light IJ, Kennan WJ, Sutherland JM: Maternal intravenous glucose administration as a cause of hypoglycemia in the infant of the diabetic mother. Am J Obstet Gynecol 113:345, 1972.
34. Pender JW, Fox M, Basso LV (eds.): Anesthesia and Uncommon Diseases. Chap. 3. Diabetes mellitus - management of the surgical patient. W.B. Saunders Co., Philadelphia, 1973.
35. Linzey EM: Controlling diabetes with continuous insulin infusion. Contemp Obstet Gynecol 12:43, 1978.
36. Steel JM, Duncan LJP, Clarke BF: Letter. Br. Med J 1:1536, 1977.
37. Felig P: Insulin: Rates and routes of delivery. N Engl J Med 291:1031, 1974.
38. Notelovitz M, Quinlan RW: Diabetes and Pregnancy - Theory and Practice. Current Problems in Obstetrics and Gynecology, III. Yearbook Medical Publishers, Chicago, 1980.
39. Felig P: Diabetic ketoacidosis. N Engl J Med 290:1360, 1974.
40. Datta S, Brown WU, Jr: Acid-base status in diabetic mothers and their infants following general or spinal anesthesia for cesarean section. Anesthesiology 47:272, 1977.
41. Datta S, et al: Epidural anesthesia for cesarean section in diabetics. Anesthesiology 51:S302, 1979.
42. Lind T, et al: Insulin disappearance rate in pregnant and non-pregnant women and in non-pregnant women given GHRIH. Eur J Clin Invest 7:47, 1977.
43. Kenepp NB, Shelley, CW, Juman S: Effects on newborn of hydration with glucose in patients undergoing cesarean section with regional anesthesia. Lancet 1:645, 1980.
44. Datta S, et al: Acid-base status of diabetic mothers and their infants following spinal anesthesia for cesarean section. Anesth Analg 61:662. 1982.
45. Mathru M, et al: Intravenous albumin administration for prevention of spinal hypotension during cesarean section. Anesth Analg 59:655, 1980.

ANESTHESIA FOR CEREBRAL VASCULAR SURGERY

J.D. MICHENFELDER, M.D.

Surgery for cerebrovascular disease can be classified into three major categories: extracranial (primarily carotid endarterectomy); intracranial (primarily aneurysms, AV malformations); and extra-intracranial anastomoses (for example superficial temporal artery to middle cerebral artery). Other than sharing the general category of cerebrovascular surgery these three types of procedures have little in common. The patients present with widely differing problems and require accordingly differing approaches for anesthetic management.

For carotid endarterectomy the major goals are to use monitoring techniques that will detect the onset of ischemia during carotid occlusion and to use anesthetic agents and techniques that will not aggravate but hopefully will prolong the brain's tolerance for such ischemia. Among various monitors recommended the most commonly used is that of stump pressure, both because it is simple and inexpensive. However, it is generally agreed that stump pressure lacks sensitivity as compared to proper monitoring of the electroencephalogram or of regional cerebral blood flow. The latter is generally not available because of both cost and complexity, although the validity of these objections may be questioned. The electroencephalogram has been condemned for the same reasons but with even less justification. Monitoring of the standard 16 lead EEG will accurately and sensitively reflect the onset of regional ischemia during carotid occlusion. In order to interpret the EEG, it must be artifact free and the patient's anesthetic depth, CO_2 levels, and brain temperature must be constant. Simplified versions of the standard EEG are now available on the market. Objections to these are either excessive cost or loss of sensitivity. It is hoped that technological progress will overcome both of these objections. Using the EEG and regional cerebral blood flow measurements it has been established in man that the critical cerebral blood flow is in the neighborhood of 18 to 24 ml/100 gm/min. In evaluating stump pressure measurement, it was found that the usually stated critical stump pressure of 50 mmHg correlated with the cerebral blood flow measurement in approximately 60 percent of the patients. In 8 percent of the patients, stump pressure was above critical levels at a time when the cerebral blood flow was below critical levels with accompanying EEG changes. With adequate monitoring the use of such controversial "protective" techniques as hypothermia or deep barbiturate anesthesia are not necessary since ischemia can be immediately recognized and corrected by the surgical insertion of a shunt during the period of carotid occlusion. Our technique of anesthesia for these patients usually includes a volatile agent, normocapnia and, during the period of carotid occlusion, a 20 percent increase in baseline cerebral perfusion pressure (if not contraindicated by cardiac pathology).

In patients undergoing surgery for aneurysms or AV malformations the major concern is usually not cerebral ischemia but rather control of blood pressure so as to avoid inadvertent rupture of the aneurysm or excessive bleeding from the AV malformation. Adequate surgical exposure is also a critical requirement thus indicating the use of techniques that will reduce brain bulk. In addition to proper anesthetic selection this may include the use of such techniques as intravenous hyperosmotic agents and drainage of cerebral spinal fluid. For induction of hypotension we currently prefer sodium nitroprusside because of both its potency and relative predictability. The concern regarding cyanide toxicity, although a real one, is easily avoided by limiting the total dose given the patient to 1 to 1.5 mg/kg. It is our clinical experience that the dose of nitroprusside required can be minimized by the use of anesthetics such as halothane or enflurane. For these patients there is no absolute contraindication to the use of induced hypotension. The risk of not using hypotension generally overrides all other risk considerations. Based upon both experimental and human work, it is reasonable to assume that a 30 percent reduction in the patient's normal blood pressure will be tolerated without any significant reduction in cerebral blood flow. If necessary, as much as a 50 percent reduction in blood pressure may be used without a major risk of cerebral ischemia although a significant reduction in cerebral blood flow will occur at these pressure levels. Greater than a 50 percent reduction in the patient's normal blood pressure may be expected to result in a time related degree of cerebral ischemia. In aneurysm surgery the major goal is to maintain a normal or reduced transmural pressure across the wall of the aneurysm. Thus before the surgeon opens the dura, a modest decrease in blood pressure should be induced since the pressure outside of the aneurysm will be abruptly decreased upon opening the dura. During manipulation of the aneurysm a 30-40 percent reduction in arterial pressure is maintained and should the aneurysm inadvertently rupture then profound degrees of hypotension may be required for the surgeon to gain control. If one anticipates the need for significant degrees of hypotension (greater than 30-40% reduction) then it would be appropriate to consider a prior dose of thiopental (3-5 mg/kg) with intermittent (every 5-10 min) small doses (½-1 mg/kg) during the period of hypotension. Hypothermia which was once the preferred technique for aneurysm surgery in many institutions has now largely been abandoned. The techniques were largely complex and time consuming and introduced complications of their own. With the introduction of the operating microscope and the use of potent hypotensive agents, the morbidity and mortality from aneurysm surgery has been greatly reduced.

For patients undergoing extracranial to intracranial vascular anastomotic procedures, the monitoring and anesthetic requirements do not normally present unusual problems. In these patients, maintenance of an adequate cerebral perfusion pressure at all times is perhaps the paramount consideration. The existing areas of cerebral ischemia for which these patients are undergoing surgery may be expected to have lost all capacity for autoregulation and thus flow to these areas is totally pressure dependent. Indeed it is not uncommon during angiographic procedures in these patients to observe transient neurologic deficits that are titratable by alterations in blood pressure. Because of the unpredictable effects of changes in CO_2 on regional cerebral blood flow in the presence of regional ischemia, we believe it is important to maintain these patients during surgery at their normal CO_2 tension. Thus we generally maintain these patients in a manner similar to that for carotid surgery. We also routinely use barbiturate therapy in these patients during the period of the actual anastomosis. Since the surgeon must temporarily occlude the branch of the middle cerebral artery to which the superficial temporal artery is being anastomosed, we assume that an unknown degree of ischemia to the area of brain supplied by that branch may occur. Therefore before surgical occlusion of the branch of the middle cerebral artery, a "sleep" dose of thiopental (3-5 mg/kg) is administered. Repeat doses are not given during the period of anastomosis since presumably if the area is ischemic we could not deliver further thiopental to it. This is an example of thiopental therapy in a situation where it will likely to no harm and may well do some good.

MANAGEMENT OF ANESTHESIA IN THE PRESENCE OF LIVER DISEASE

ROBERT K. STOELTING, M.D.

Management of anesthesia in the presence of liver disease requires an understanding of the 1) physiologic functions of the liver 2) determinants of hepatic blood flow and 3) significance of liver function tests.

PHYSIOLOGIC FUNCTIONS OF THE LIVER

Glucose Homeostasis

The liver is essential for maintenance of normal blood glucose levels particularly during the fasting state introduced before elective operation. This is accomplished by storage of glucose in the hepatocyte as glycogen. Breakdown of glycogen (glycogenolysis) releases glucose back into the systemic circulation. In addition, glycerol from adipose tissue, amino acids from skeletal muscle and lactate produced by normal metabolism in erythrocytes and skeletal muscle or during low flow states, may be converted to glucose (gluconeogenesis) in the liver. Metabolic acidosis in the patient with liver disease may reflect the inability of the damaged liver to convert lactic acid to glucose. Furthermore, chronic liver disease may be associated with glycogen depletion which can predispose to hypoglycemia particularly during the perioperative period.
An understanding of bilirubin formation and elimination is important for differentiating intrahepatic from prehepatic or posthepatic dysfunction.

Protein synthesis

Drug binding. All proteins, except gamma globulins, are synthesized in the liver. Liver disease may result in decreased albumin production such that fewer sites are available for drug binding. As a result, the unbound pharmacologically active drug fraction increases and unexpected drug sensitivities may occur. In contrast, resistance to the effects of d-tubocurarine has been observed in patients with cirrhosis. This resistance may reflect increased d-tubocurarine binding to gamma globulin, sequestration in inactive tissue sites, or increased distribution volume due to circulatory changes (increased cardiac output) associated with chronic liver disease.

Recent data have demonstrated prolonged plasma half-times, decreased plasma clearance and increased distribution volume for pancuronium in patients with alcoholic cirrhosis (1). Based on these observations, it is conceivable the initial dose of pancuronium necessary to produce adequate muscle relaxation might be increased because the drug is diluted in a large distribution volume while the duration of paralysis would be prolonged due to slowed plasma clearance.

Coagulation. Severe liver disease must occur before impaired coagulation is manifest. This is related to the fact that many coagulation factors require only 30 percent of normal activity for adequate clotting to occur. Nevertheless, the plasma half-times of hepatic produced clotting factors, including prothrombin and fibrinogen, are brief and acute liver dysfunction is likely to be associated with clotting abnormalities.

Decreased prothrombin production may reflect severe hepatocellular disease or impaired vitamin K absorption due to biliary obstruction and absence of bile salts. Parenteral vitamin K restores prothrombin production due to biliary obstruction but may not be effective if hepatocellular disease is severe.

Cholinesterase activity. Another protein whose production is impaired by liver disease is cholinesterase (pseudocholinesterase). A fourfold reduction in cholinesterase activity in association with liver disease increased slightly the duration of apnea following succinylcholine (2). Nevertheless, prolonged apnea (greater than 1 hour) is unlikely from liver disease alone and atypical cholinesterase enzyme must be suspected. The half-time of cholinesterase is about 14 days such that acute liver failure is unlikely to alter the rate of succinylcholine hydrolysis.

Drug biotransformation

Chronic liver disease may result in decreased microsomal enzyme activity and slowed drug metabolism. Indeed, prolonged plasma half-times for diazepam, meperidine, and lidocaine, as well as increased barbiturate sleep time, have been demonstrated in patients with cirrhosis. In contrast, the alcoholic patient may manifest resistance to drugs metabolized in the liver reflecting microsomal enzyme induction from chronic ethanol ingestion and/or cellular tolerance to depressant drugs.

HEPATIC BLOOD FLOW

The liver receives approximately 25 percent of the cardiac output via the hepatic artery (20-40 percent of the total flow) and portal vein. Anesthetic drugs as well as regional anesthesia reduce hepatic blood flow (HBF) 20-30 percent. These changes reflect effects on perfusion pressure and/or splanchnic vascular resistance. Surgical stimulation may further decrease HBF with the greatest reductions occurring during intra-abdominal operations (3).

A potential adverse effect produced by decreased HBF is decreased oxygen delivery and resulting hepatocyte hypoxia. Hepatocyte hypoxia may have implications with respect to metabolism of anesthetics. Specifically, low hepatocyte oxygen concentrations may favor reductive (anaerobic) metabolism. To date, however, reductive metabolism has been demonstrated to occu only with halothane. Since reductive metabolites of halothane are potentially hepatotoxic, maintenance of hepatic oxygenation via an adequate HBF during anesthesia has special significance.

Reductions in HBF will also reduce drug delivery to the liver for biotransformation resulting in increased drug effects. Drugs with high hepatic extraction ratios, such as lidocaine or propranolol, will be particularly influenced. This is the reason that lower doses of lidocaine may be required during anesthesia to achieve blood levels similar to those in the awake state.

LIVER FUNCTION TESTS

Liver function tests permit classification of hepatic dysfunction as prehepatic, intrahepatic and posthepatic (Table). It is important to remember that liver function tests are rarely specific and considerable damage must be present before values are altered. Furthermore, liver disease may produce little alteration in function and only when some additional insult (operation) produces further deterioration does the underlying liver disease become obvious.

Table

	BILIRUBIN	TRANSAMINASES	ALKALINE PHOSPHATASE
PREHEPATIC	Increased Unconjugated Fraction	Normal	Normal
INTRAHEPATIC	Increased Conjugated Fraction	Elevated	Normal
POSTHEPATIC	Increased Conjugated Fraction	Normal	Elevated

Postoperatively, the magnitude of liver dysfunction as reflected by liver function tests is exaggerated by operations near the liver. There is no evidence that the specific anesthetic drug influences the magnitude of postoperative liver dysfunction as reflected by these tests. Furthermore, regardless of the operative site, postoperative liver dysfunction is accentuated in the patient with preexisting liver disease.

Serum bilirubin

Protein bound (indirect) bilirubin cannot be excreted by the kidneys while conjugated (direct) bilirubin may appear in the urine. Overt jaundice is present when serum bilirubin exceeds 3 mg/100 ml (normal less than 1 mg/100 ml) but there may be no correlation between the level of serum bilirubin and the severity of liver disease.

Serum transaminases (SGOT, SGPT, LDH)

Hepatocytes contain large amounts of the transaminase enzymes such that acute hepatocellular damage (hypoxia, drugs, viral hepatitis) causes these substances to spill into the systemic circulation. Other tissues such as heart, lung and skeletal muscle, contain these enzymes emphasizing that elevations may not be specific for liver damage. It is important to remember that serum transaminases (especially SGOT) may be elevated during the asymptomatic prodromal phase of viral hepatitis.

Serum alkaline phosphatase

This enzyme is present in bile duct cells and when elevated distinguishes obstructive from hepatocellular disease. Skeletal muscle also contains large amounts of alkaline phosphatase.

Serum albumin

An albumin concentration below 3.5 gms/100 ml signifies severe cirrhosis. Indeed, patients with low serum albumin concentrations are most likely to manifest altered drug responses due to decreased protein binding and/or biotransformation. The half-time for albumin is about 23 days such that acute liver dysfunction may not be reflected by decreased serum albumin levels Albumin/globulin ratios have little significance as a measure of liver function since globulin does not depend on hepatic synthesis

ANESTHESIA FOR PATIENTS WITH LIVER DISEASE

The management of anesthesia in the presence of liver disease is based on an understanding of the pathophysiological changes associated with chronic liver disease. The best anesthetic drug choice or technique in the presence of liver disease is not known. However, it is important to remember that a constant feature of chronic liver disease is decreased HBF due to increased resistance to flow through the portal vein. This reduced HBF has implications for hepatocyte oxygenation. Furthermore, postoperative liver dysfunction is likely to be exaggerated in any patient with chronic liver dysfunction regardless of the anesthetic drug administered.

The administration of halothane to a patient with known liver disease poses a dilemma. There is no data that demonstrates halothane accentuates underlying liver disease. Nevertheless, factors that favor reductive metabolism of halothane may be more likely to be present in the patient with liver disease (especially ethanol produced) than in a normal patient. Specifically, chronic ethanol abuse may induce hepatic microsomal enzymes while fibrotic parenchymal changes characteristic of cirrhosis predictably decrease HBF and jeopardize hepatocyte oxygenation. Anesthetic drugs and surgical stimulation may even further decrease HBF. The theoretical hazard of enzyme induction and hepatocyte hypoxia secondary to reductions in HBF is emphasized by the animal models for halothane hepatotoxicity (4). On the basis of these animal data and the changes known to predictably occur in the patient with chronic liver disease, the choice of halothane for maintenance of anesthesia may be questionable particularly when alternative drugs such as enflurane or isoflurane are available.

In addition to altered responses to thiobarbiturates and neuromuscular blockers, it is a clinical impression that requirements for inhaled anesthetics are increased in patients who chronically abuse ethanol. This impression is supported by the observation that mice exposed to alcohol manifest increased isoflurane requirements. In man, halothane MAC in alcoholic patients was 1 percent compared with 0.75 percent in normal patients.

Liver disease is associated with increased venous admixture reflecting the presence of portosystemic and intrapulmonary shunts. These shunts develop in response to the increased resistance to blood flow through the diseased liver. Vasodilation from inhaled or injected anesthetics may increase the magnitude of right-to-left shunt and further reduce arterial oxygenation.

Cirrhosis may result in decreased glycogen stores such that hypoglycemia may occur intraoperatively if exogenous glucose is not provided.

The hepatorenal syndrome is renal failure seen in association with liver disease. Typically, this occurs in patients with alcoholic cirrhosis. The incidence of postoperative renal failure is also increased in patients with obstructive jaundice. Data suggest that renal failure in these patients may be minimized by intraoperative antibiotics and maintenance of intraoperative diuresis with 5 percent mannitol.

REFERENCES

1. Duvaldstein P, Agostin S, Henzel D, Kerstein UN, Desmonts JM. Pancuronium pharmacokinetics in patients with liver cirrhosis Br J Anaesth 1979;50:1131-6.
2. Foldes FF, Swerdlow M, Kipschitz E, et al. Comparison of the respiratory effects of suxamethonium and suxethonium in man. Anesthesiology 1956;17:559-63.
3. Gelman SI. Disturbances in hepatic blood flow during anesthesia and surgery. Arch Surg 1976;111:881-4.
4. Widger LA, Gandolfi AJ, Van Dyke RA. Hypoxia and halothane metabolism in vivo: Release of inorganic fluoride and halothane metabolite binding to cellular constituents. Anesthesiology 1976;44:197-201.

SPECIAL TECHNIQUES IN NEUROANESTHESIA

J.D. MICHENFELDER, M.D.

I. Choice of Anesthetic Agents and Techniques
   A. If intracranial pressure is the major concern:
      1. Avoid when possible volatile anesthetics
      2. Select intravenous agents (except for ketamine)
         a. Narcotic + relaxant ± N_2O is excellent choice (neuroleptic is optional)
         b. Thiopental infusion is theoretically acceptable but results in post-op depression
   B. In certain circumstances, volatile agents (halothane or enflurane) may be desirable or indicated:
      1. If N_2O is contraindicated
         a. Following air contrast studies
         b. If air embolism is likely
      2. If stable controlled BP is required or hypotension is to be induced
      3. Use volatile agents in lowest possible concentration
      4. Always hyperventilate ($PaCO_2$ 25-30 torr) preferably prior to introducing agent
   C. Pay close attention to details of good technique during induction
      1. Avoid anxiety inducing actions
         a. Premature placement of face mask
         b. Over-vigorous pre-oxygenation
      2. Barbiturate induction is usually indicated
      3. Avoid extreme flexion, extension, or rotation of head
      4. Guarantee adequate paralysis - block-aid monitor
      5. Guarantee adequate anesthetic depth (induce surgical levels of anesthesia)
      6. Then intubate
   D. If intracranial pressure increases are to be prevented, you must

avoid when possible:

1. Volatile agents
2. Hypercapnia
3. Increase in venous pressure
4. Increase in arterial pressure
5. Inadequate relaxation
6. Respiratory obstruction
7. Excessive fluid therapy
8. Improper fluid therapy (avoid dextrose in H_2O)
9. Sympathetic stimulation

E. Hazards of increased intracranial pressure
   1. Decrease in cerebral perfusion pressure (global)
      a. CPP = MAP - ICP
      b. Maintain CPP above 40-50 mm in normotensive patients
      c. Higher CPP required in hypertensive patients
   2. Regional decreases in CBF
      a. Pathologic areas do not autoregulate and flow is pressure dependent
   3. Herniation of brain through fixed structures with brain stem compression

II. Special techniques for reducing brain bulk

A. Osmotic agents
   1. Dosage + timing are important - the more rapidly administered, the smaller the dose
   2. Initially circulating volume expansion, followed by diuresis and volume contraction
   3. Rebound occurs; urea > mannitol
   4. Avoid infiltration or administration into a relatively static venous bed

B. Diuretic
   1. A reasonable alternative to osmotic agents
   2. Fewer side effects
   3. Probably not as effective in reducing brain bulk

C. Lumbar CSF drainage
   1. Hazardous in presence of increased ICP
   2. Effective in neurovascular and pituitary surgery

D. Cortisone

1. Controversial
2. Perhaps useful in chronic RX

III. Special considerations in posterior fossa surgery (sitting position)

A. Postural hypotension (prevention and management)
   1. Light anesthesia
   2. Consider volume load before positioning
   3. Compress dependent venous bed (elastic bandages, Gardner G-suit)
   4. Use semi-reclining rather than true sitting position
   5. Think in terms of pressure <u>at head level</u>
   6. Use vasopressors to RX <u>any</u> fall in BP

B. Air embolism (prevention and management)
   1. Monitoring
      a. Esophageal stethoscope
      b. Doppler
      c. Right atrial catheter
      d. Expired CO_2
      e. Plus routine (EKG, BP, etc.)
   2. Etiology
      a. Whenever the height of the surgical wound above the heart (in cm) exceeds the venous pressure (in cm in H_2O), the potential for air embolism exists
      b. When potential exists, an open vein must either collapse or aspirate air
      c. In the posterior fossa there are many non-collapsible veins (diploic veins and dural sinuses)
   3. Prevention
      a. Maintain adequate circulating volume
      b. Control ventilation
      c. Careful surgical technique
   4. Diagnosis
      a. Doppler sound changes most sensitive
      b. Cardiac murmur (characteristic for air)
      c. Decrease in expired CO_2
      d. Arrhythmias
      e. Hypotension
      f. Miscellaneous
      g. Confirmed by aspiration of air from right atrium

5. RX
    a. Increase venous pressure in wound
        1) jugular compression (bilateral)
        2) PEEP
        3) lower head
    b. Remove air from heart
        1) aspirate atrial catheter
        2) maintain or stimulate cardiac contractility
    c. DC N_2O
    d. Symptomatic

IV. Monitoring brain stem function
  A. Traditionally neurosurgeons monitor spontaneous ventilation
    1. Change in rate, rhythm, or volume signals untoward brain stem stimulation
    2. Disadvantages include hypercarbia, hypertension, increased potential for air embolism, deeper levels of anesthesia
  B. Alternative is to monitor for sudden alterations in cardiac rate and rhythm
    1. Appears to be equally sensitive to monitoring respiration
    2. Permits use of controlled ventilation
    3. Avoid RX of arrhythmias if possible - otherwise may mask that which you are monitoring

V. Monitoring cortical function
  A. Manifestations of cerebral function
    1. Regional anesthesia - observe neurologic function
    2. EEG
        a. Anesthetic depth must be light and steady
        b. $PaCO_2$ must be known and steady
        c. Must be constantly attended
        d. Not practical during most craniotomies
    3. Vital signs
        a. Good indicator of brain stem function not cortical function
  B. Cerebral metabolic events
    1. Jugular bulb blood O_2 levels
        a. Do not reflect regional events
        b. May be misleading
    2. Blood or CSF lactate levels

a. Late manifestation of ischemia

C. CBF

1. Complex and usually impractical
2. Subject to inaccuracy
3. Must know $PaCO_2$
4. Regional information superior to average whole brain measurements

D. Cerebral perfusion pressure

1. Technically need both MAP and ICP
2. MAP adequate if dura opened
3. "Stump" pressure may be used in carotid surgery
4. Pressure alone does not necessarily reflect flow

E. Evoked response

1. Promising development
2. As yet not technically practical

REFERENCES

1. Plum F, Siesjo B: Recent advances in CSF physiology. Anesthesiology 41:708, 1975.
2. Larson CP, et al: Effect of anesthetics on cerebral, renal and splanchnic circulations: Recent developments. Anesthesiology 41:169, 1974.
3. Fink BR, Haschke RH: Anesthetic effects on cerebral metabolism. Anesthesiology 39:199, 1973.
4. Smith A, Wollman H: Cerebral blood flow and metabolism: Effects of anesthetic drugs and techniques. Anesthesiology 36:378, 1972.
5. Alexander SC, Lassen NA: Cerebral circulatory response to acute brain disease: Implications for anesthetic practice. Anesthesiology 32:60, 1970.
6. Michenfelder JD, et al: Neuroanesthesia. Anesthesiology 30:65, 1969.

CHANGING CONCEPTS IN PREANESTHETIC MEDICATION

ROBERT K. STOELTING, M.D.

Anesthetic management begins with the preoperative psychological preparation of the patient and administration of a drug or drugs selected to produce specific pharmacologic responses prior to the induction of anesthesia. Traditionally, this initial psychological and pharmacological component of anesthetic management is referred to as preanesthetic medication.

PREOPERATIVE PSYCHOLOGICAL PREPARATION

The psychological component of preoperative preparation is provided by the anesthesiologist's visit and interview. The value of this interview is evidenced by its demonstrable calming effect (Table 1) (1).

Table 1.

	PERCENT OF PATIENTS	
	INTERVIEW	PENTOBARBITAL*
FEEL NERVOUS	40%	61%
FEEL DROWSY	26%	30%
JUDGED SEDATED	65%	48%

*2 mg/kg intramuscularly 1 hour before surgery

PREOPERATIVE PHARMACOLOGIC PREPARATION

The most important objective of preoperative pharmacologic preparation is anxiety relief. Ideally, patients should enter the preoperative period free from apprehension, sedated but easily arousable and fully cooperative. Other goals may include analgesia, amnesia, reduction of salivary gland and gastric fluid secretions, elevation of gastric fluid pH, and decreased cardiac vagal activity. No drug or drug combination achieves all these goals. After a thorough evaluation of the patient, it may be appropriate not to include drugs in the preoperative preparation.

Drugs likely to be considered for administration as preanesthetic medication include barbiturates, narcotics, tranquilizers, anticholinergics and histamine H_2 receptor antagonists.

Barbiturates

Secobarbital and pentobarbital are examples of barbiturates used for preoperative medication. Advantages cited for these drugs include sedation, minimal respiratory depressant effects, minimal circulatory depression, rarity of nausea and vomiting and effectiveness when administered orally. Disadvantages include lack of analgesia, disorientation especially if administered to patients in pain and absence of a specific pharmacologic antagonist.

Narcotics

Morphine and meperidine are the narcotics most frequently used. Fentanyl does not have an appropriate onset and duration of action to justify recommending its use as preoperative medication. Adverse side effects of narcotics include relaxation of peripheral vascular smooth muscle manifesting as orthostatic hypotension. In contrast to barbiturates, narcotics used for preoperative medication depress the medullary respiratory center. The euphoric effect of narcotics in patients with pain may be dysphoria in the absence of pain. Nausea and vomiting have been attributed to a specific narcotic effect on the vestibular apparatus or stimulation of the chemoreceptor trigger zone. Narcotic-induced smooth muscle constriction may be manifest as choledochoduodenal sphincter spasm causing some to question the use of narcotics in patients with biliary tract disease.

Tranquilizers

Diazepam and lorazepam are considered to be specific for anxiety relief. In addition, vomiting and significant cardiorespiratory depression do not occur. Disadvantages may include discomfort at the injection site following intramuscular or intravenous administration and prolonged duration of action. In animals, diazepam increases the seizure threshold for lidocaine but there is no evidence in man that diazepam used as preoperative medication reduces the likelihood of local anesthetic toxicity (2).

Droperidol is used for anxiety relief and is a potent antiemetic. A major disadvantage is the occasional patient who develops acute anxiety following droperidol. In addition, this drug is a dopaminergic receptor blocker and may produce extrapyramidal symptoms particularly in patients with paralysis agitans.

Hydroxyzine and promethazine manifest antihistaminic, antiemetic and sedative properties. These drugs may add to the sedative effects of narcotics without producing additional respiratory depression.

Anticholinergics

Atropine, scopolamine and glycopyrrolate are examples of anticholinergics used in preoperative medication. Atropine and scopolamine are tertiary amines and can cross lipid barriers such as the blood brain barrier, placenta and gastrointestinal tract. In contrast, glycopyrrolate acts only on peripheral cholinergic receptors as its quaternary ammonium structure prevents it from crossing lipid barriers in significant amounts.

Antisialagogue effect. The need for including an anticholinergic in the preoperative medication to produce an antisialagogue effect has been questioned since currently used inhaled anesthetics do not stimulate excessive upper airway secretions. Nevertheless, more satisfactory conditions during general anesthesia due to decreased secretions are likely when an anticholinergic is administered preoperatively (3). An antisialagogue is particularly important for intraoral operations or when topical anesthesia is necessary as excessive secretions may interfere with the surgery or impair production of topical anesthesia by diluting the local anesthetic. As an antisialagogue glycopyrrolate is more potent and longer lasting than glycopyrrolate.

Production of sedative and amnesic effects. Scopolamine produces useful sedative effects particularly in combination with other drugs used for preoperative medication. Scopolamine is 8-9 times more potent than atropine in this respect. Sedative effects following glycopyrrolate would be unlikely.

Decreased gastric hydrogen ion secretion. The value of an anticholinergic in elevating gastric fluid pH is questionable. Atropine or glycopyrrolate administered intramuscularly 1 to 1.5 hours before induction of anesthesia in adult patients is not effective in significantly raising gastric fluid pH or reducing gastric fluid volume as compared with patients not receiving an anticholinergic (4).

Prevention of reflex bradycardia. Prevention of reflex bradycardia seems unlikely with the timing and dose of intramuscular anticholinergic typically administered for preoperative medication. If an anticholinergic is selected to prevent reflex bradycardia, the most logical approach is to administer atropine or glycopyrrolate intravenously shortly before the anticipated need.

Central nervous system toxicity. The central anticholinergic syndrome represents toxic central nervous system effects of anticholinergics. Symptoms include restlessness, agitation and prolonged somnolence after anesthesia. Toxicity is more likely to follow scopolamine than atropine but the incidence should be low with the doses used for preoperative medication. Nevertheless, elderly patients may be particularly susceptible to central toxic effects from both drugs. A central anticholinergic syndrome after glycopyrrolate is unlikely.

Relaxation of the lower esophageal sphincter. Atropine, scopolamine and glycopyrrolate in doses used for preoperative medication decrease the resting tone of the lower esophageal sphincter. Conceivably, reduction in sphincter tone could increase the risk of gastroesophageal reflux.

Heart rate changes. Theoretically, heart rate may increase after intramuscular anticholinergic administration. When an increased heart rate would be undesirable, the use of scopolamine or glycopyrrolate is least likely to increase heart rate. Nevertheless, the most likely cardiac response after intramuscula atropine as used in preoperative medication is heart rate slowing

Mydriasis and cycloplegia. Atropine and scopolamine may produce mydriasis and cycloplegia such that patients may experience visual impairment postoperatively. Scopolamine has a greater mydriatic effect than atropine. Despite the drug-induced mydriasis, an anticholinergic may be safely included in the preoperative medication of a patient with glaucoma.

Histamine H2-receptor antagonist

Cimetidine is a histamine H2-receptor antagonist that counters the ability of histamine to induce secretion of gastric fluid with a high hydrogen ion concentration. Therefore, this drug offers a pharmacologic approach for increasing gastric fluid pH preoperatively. Indeed, oral cimetidine (300 mg) administered to adult patients 1 to 1.5 hours before induction of anesthesia increases the gastric fluid pH above 2.5 in over 80 percent of patients (Table 2) (5). It must be appreciated that cimetidine prolongs the elimination half-time of diazepam but not lorazepam. Cimetidine may also increase airway resistanc in patients with obstructive pulmonary disease.

Preoperative antacids also increase gastric fluid pH at the time of anesthetic induction but in contrast to cimetidine increase gastric fluid volume. Furthermore, antacids may have adverse effects on the tracheobronchial tree if they are aspirated. In the future, metoclopramide may be appropriate for administration to selected patients to facilitate emptying of the stomach prior to induction of anesthesia.

Table 2. PERCENT OF PATIENTS WITH GASTRIC FLUID pH SAMPLES (5)

PREOPERATIVE MEDICATION	BELOW 2.5	2.5-5.0	ABOVE 5
MORPHINE ATROPINE	60%	34%	6%
MORPHINE ATROPINE CIMETIDINE*	16%**	24%	60%**

*300 mg orally 1 to 1.5 hours before induction of anesthesia

**P < 0.05 compared with morphine-atropine

RECOMMENDED APPROACH TO PREOPERATIVE MEDICATION

Preanesthetic medication is most appropriately administered 1 to 2 hours before induction of anesthesia. Intramuscular injections are unpleasant such that oral administration is ideal. Oral cimetidine is also conveniently administered at this time. The small amount of water (30-45 ml) needed for oral administration of drugs is negligible with respect to gastric fluid volume. If pain is present preoperatively or preparation for anesthesia is likely to be uncomfortable (invasive monitoring, nerve blocks), an intramuscular narcotic is indicated.

Intramuscular administration of scopolamine at the same time as the oral drugs or intramuscular narcotic is indicated when one wishes to exploit the amnesic and sedative effects of this anticholinergic. The combination of intramuscular morphine and scopolamine is ideal for producing tranquility and sedation in patients most deserving of aggressive pharmacologic preoperative medication.

An anticholinergic selected to produce an antisialagogue effect is most appropriately administered intramuscularly immediately before the patient is sent to the operating room. If the anticholinergic is given 1 to 2 hours before induction of anesthesia, the patient is more likely to be uncomfortable from a dry mouth. Glycopyrrolate is the most logical drug if an antisialagogue response without central nervous system effects is desired.

REFERENCES

1. Egbert LD, Battit GE, Turndorf H, et al. The value of the preoperative visit by an anesthetist. JAMA 1963;185:553-5.
2. Moore DC, Balfour RI, Fitzgibbons D. Convulsive arterial plasma levels of bupivacaine and the response to diazepam therapy. Anesthesiology 1979;50:454-6.
3. Falick YS, Smiler BG. Is anticholinergic premedication necessary? Anesthesiology 1975;43:472-3.
4. Stoelting RK. Responses to atropine, glycopyrrolate, and Riopan of gastric fluid pH and volume in adult patients. Anesthesiology 1978;48:367-9.
5. Stoelting RK. Gastric fluid pH in patients receiving cimetidine. Anesth Analg 1978;57:675-7.

CALCIUM CHANNEL BLOCKERS AND ANESTHESIA

J.G. REVES

The purpose of this report is to examine the interaction of anesthetic drugs with calcium channel blockers. This is an area of intensive investigation at several centers. We have recently reviewed the pharmacology of nifedipine and verapamil, and their implications in the practice of anesthesiology (1). Diltiazem will be available in the United States soon and McAuley and Schroeder have written an excellent review of its pharmacology (2). For other review articles on this subject I recommend references 3-7. Tables 1 and 2 contain comparisons of interest to anesthesiologists concerning the three Ca^{++} entry blockers.

Table 1.
PHARMACOLOGIC CHARACTERISTICS OF CALCIUM CHANNEL BLOCKERS

	NIFEDIPINE	VERAPAMIL	DILTIAZEM
Dosage			
oral	10-20 mg t.i.d.	80-160 mg t.i.d.	40-80 mg t.i.d.
i.v.	5-15 μg/kg	150 μg/kg	15-30 μg/kg
Absorption			
oral (%)	> 90	> 90	> 90
bioaval (%)	65-70+	10-20	?
Onset Action			
oral (min)	< 20	< 30	< 30
subl (min)	3	-	-
i.v. (min)	1-3	1-3	-
Protein Binding (%)	90	90	80-85%
Elimination t½ (hr)	5	2-7*	4-6
Active metabolites	no ?	yes	
Excretion			
renal (%)	80	70	35
fecal (%)	< 15	15	65

Where Bioaval = bioavailability, subl = sublingual, + nifedipine is light sensitive and should be protected from light, * = normal patients (5,8-10)

Table 2.

COMPARISON OF CARDIOVASCULAR EFFECTS CALCIUM CHANNEL BLOCKERS

	NIFEDIPINE	VERAPAMIL	DILTIAZEM
Systemic Vasodilation	++	+	+
A-V Conduction Slowing	-	++	+
Negative Inotropism	-	+	-

<u>Background</u>

General anesthetics as a group are cardiovascular depressants and it is now fairly well established that the myocardial depression (11-13) and vascular dilation (14) are at least in part related to interference with movement and/or translocation of Ca^{++} across membranes and intracellularly. The negative inotropic effects of halothane are not fully understood but appear to be related to changes in intracellular Ca^{++} kinetics (12,15). Halothane and enflurane prolong A-V conduction (16-18), halothane in part by Ca^{++} channel blockade (19). There is considerable potential then for drug interactions related to the cardiovascular system between general anesthetic drugs and Ca^{++} channel blockers.

<u>Laboratory Reports</u>

Kapur and coworkers have done a great deal of work examining the interaction of <u>verapamil</u> and various inhalation anesthetics. They showed that in the intact dog, verapamil (0.2 mg/kg i.v. over 30 sec) produced transient but significant decreases in SVR, blood pressure, LV dP/dt, and increases in LVEDP, cardiac output and P-R interval in dogs anesthetized with 1.1 MAC halothane. Except for the P-R interval, these changes were brief, generally returning toward control in 10-20 minutes. The cardiovascular changes could be minimized by giving the same dose over a longer time period (20). They have also shown that the administration of verapamil during isoflurane and enflurane produces hemodynamic consequences qualitatively similar to those during halothane, but infusion of verapamil produces less hemodynamic depression during 1 MAC isoflurane than 1 MAC enflurane (21). Kates and coworkers employed a right heart bypass technic and found that when afterload is kept constant, dose related decreases in left ventricular function occur with the combination of verapamil and isoflurane (22). A potential serious drug interaction of inhalation anesthetics with verapamil is the potential development of A-V block, since both drugs significantly prolong A-V conduction (18,20,23) and reversal of block is difficult. If verapamil plus enflurane, isoflurane or halothane combinations are used the P-R interval should be monitored carefully.

Although verapamil is not the drug of choice for ventricular arrhythmias, Kapur and Flacke have demonstrated the antiarrhythmic effect of verapamil (.2 mg/kg i.v.) on epinephrine induced ventricular arrhythmias in halothane (.9%) anesthetized dogs. Verapamil produced cumulative dose related increases in the arrhythmogenic dose of epinephrine. I believe lidocaine is a more appropriate drug in the clinical equivalent of this study; nevertheless, the antiarrhythmic effect of verapamil in epinephrine induced arrhythmias is clearly established in the work of Kapur and Flacke (24).

Another potential drug interaction is with verapamil and neuromuscular blocking agents. Kraynack and collaborators found that relatively high doses of verapamil diminish the muscle twitch amplitude of the pentobarbital anesthetized cat (25). The mechanism for this action is unclear, but probably involves some non Ca^{++} entry blocking properties of verapamil. The clinical significance of verapamil's action on skeletal muscle and interaction with neuromuscular blockers need's further study.

Tosone in our laboratory has investigated the interaction of nifedipine (10-15 µg/kg i.v. over 2 minutes) and halothane in normal dogs and found that there is an initial decrease in SVR, blood pressure, cardiac output, left ventricular dP/dt and contractile force after nifedipine administration which by 30 minutes is not significantly different from baseline 1% or 2% halothane (26). The acute administration of nifedipine (10 µg/kg) to the intact halothane anesthetized dog produces significant decreases in mean arterial pressure which is mostly a result of decreased systemic vascular resistance. The response is greater in dogs anesthetized with 2% halothane than 1% (27). Marshall also working in our laboratory employed isolated perfused rat hearts to examine the interaction of nifedipine and halothane on myocardial contractility (dP/dt) and peak systolic tension (PLV). Within clinical dose ranges, he found that the direct negative inotropic effects of nifedipine and halothane are mostly additive (Fig. 1). The clinical implications of these laboratory investigations are that in normal man the cardiovascular depression of inhalation anesthetics and nifedipine are probably close to being additive; therefore, lower doses of each should be initially given, but that the combination is probably safe.

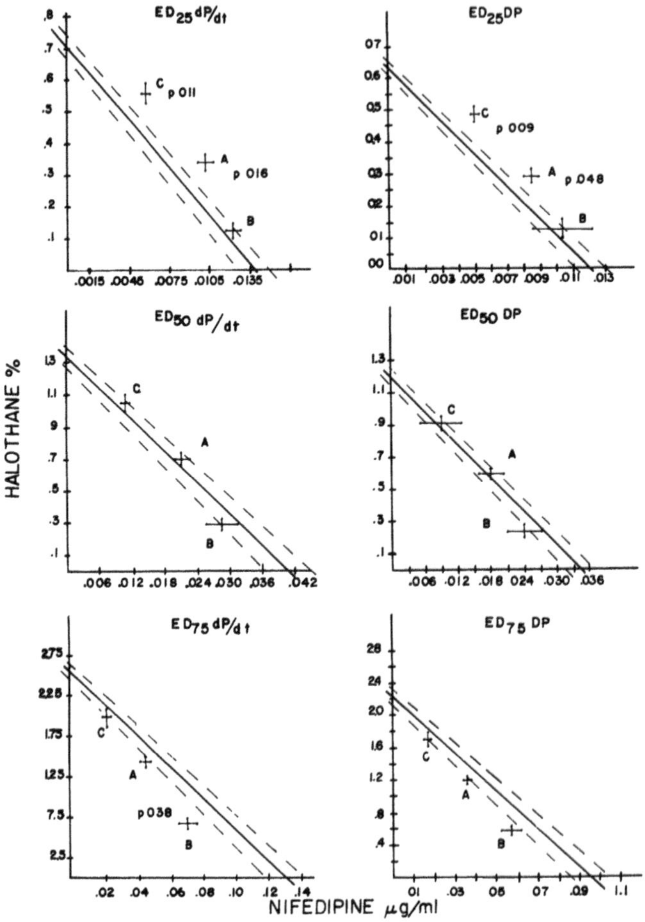

FIGURE 1. Isobolographic analysis showing the interaction of halothane and nifedipine on two indices of myocardial contractility, the dP/dt and the developed tension (DP). In each panel the negative inotropic effects of halothane alone and nifedipine alone are plotted and joined by the dark line with standard error of the mean as broken lines. This constitutes the isobol. These isobols are drawn at three conditions 25%, 50%, and 75% myocardial depression (ED_{25}, ED_{50}, ED_{75}). Points A, B, and C on each graph represent combinations of halothane:nifedipine in potency ratios of 1:1 (group A) 1:3 (group B) and 3:1 (group C). Note that at ED_{25} most combinations of halothane and nifedipine either lie along the additive line or above it suggesting that the combination of halothane and nifedipine with low levels of myocardial depression is additive or infra-additive. At ED_{50} the combinations of halothane and nifedipine fall within the additive dose field showing that halothane and nifedipine with moderate depression act in an additive way. Finally, at ED_{75} there is a slight suggestion that combinations of halothane and nifedipine appear to be additive or slightly supra-additive. The conclusion from this data is that in usual dose ranges of nifedipine and halothane we would expect additive negative inotropic effects as seen in the ED_{50} panels.

Human Reports

In man there is only limited information regarding the interaction of Ca^{++} entry blockers and anesthesia. In a large series of patients "lightly anesthetized" with halothane, verapamil in large doses (up to 20 mg i.v.) was given safely (23), but decreases in blood pressure of 5 minute duration and a 4% incidence of increased P-R interval occurred. We examined anesthesia in nifedipine treated patients in a study involving thirty-two patients electively scheduled for coronary artery bypass surgery. Seven patients (Group N) were chronically maintained on nifedipine 40 to 80 mg daily for treatment of angina pectoris. Nifedipine was discontinued the night before operation. The 25 other patients (Group C) served as a control group. Patients were on similar doses of propranolol, isosorbide dinitrate, and nitroglycerin for treatment of their heart disease. A radial arterial catheter was placed for continuous measurement of arterial systolic and diastolic blood pressure (SBP/DBP). Heart rate, rhythm and ST segment configurations were continuously monitored with the V_5 electrocardiogram. Anesthesia was induced with diazepam .3-.5 mg/kg followed by N_2O/O_2 50:50, pancuronium .1 mg/kg, and enflurane .5-2%. Hemodynamic measurements were recorded in both groups at the following intervals: 1) control (baseline before induction), 2) after intubation 3) at nadir of hemodynamic changes during surgical preparation of patient, and 4) at zenith of hemodynamic changes after sternotomy.

Table 3 contains the hemodynamic data for both groups and the rate pressure product for each group is in Fig. 2. There were no ST changes indicative of myocardial ischemia in any of the patients at each of the intervals. The hemodynamic response in both groups are similar at most stressful periods: intubation produced the most marked hemodynamic changes, 25% and 23% increases in SBP in Group N and C, respectively. The diastolic blood pressure fell below 60 torr in 2 patients in Group N and phenylephrine was given as N_2O/enflurane were discontinued to correct the hypotension. Heart rate responses tended to be more variable in Group C than Group N, but RPP changes were similar in both groups except during prep where they were lower in Group N (Fig. 2).

TABLE 3:
HEMODYNAMIC CHANGES AT VARIOUS TIMES DURING ANESTHESIA FOR CABG

	CONTROL		INTUBATION	
	N	C	N	C
SBP	141 ± 9.7	132 ± 4.8	176 ± 8.8	163 ± 5.3
DBP	75 ± 2.7	80 ± 2.3	94 ± 4.9	92 ± 3.8
HR	76 ± 4.9	72 ± 1.8	80 ± 4.9	91 ± 4.3
	PREP		**STERNOTOMY**	
	N	C	N	C
SBP	103 ± 9.6	116 ± 3.3	159 ± 20.6	140 ± 5.6
DBP	60 ± 6.2+	71 ± 2.4	85 ± 8.6	86 ± 3.7
HR	67 ± 2.2*	74 ± 2.5	68 ± 2.2	76 ± 3.0

Where N = nifedipine group (n = 7), C = control group (n = 25), * $p < .05$ N vs C, + 2 patients were given brief infusion of phenylephrine to raise the DBP > 60 torr.

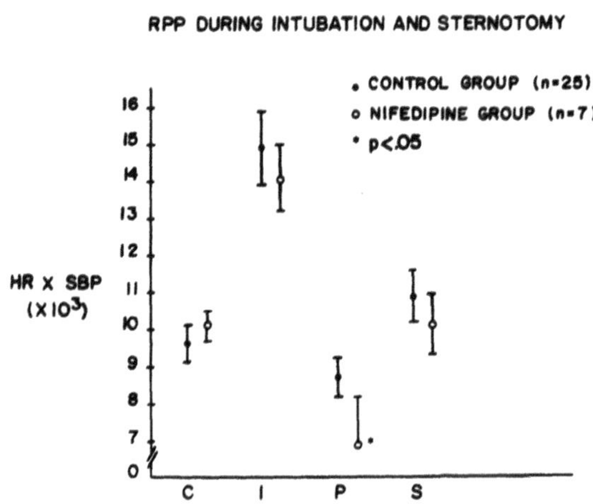

FIGURE 2. Rate pressure product observed in patients not treated with nifedipine (control group) and in those maintained on nifedipine (nifedipine group). Where C = control (prior to anesthesia induction), I = intubation, P = surgical prep (no stimulation) and S = sternotomy. The only significant difference in these groups occurs during prep when the rate pressure product is lower in the nifedipine group.

These data demonstrate that patients maintained on their nifedipine until the evening before surgery behave in a similar fashion to those not taking nifedipine when anesthetized with diazepam, N_2O, and enflurane. The exception to this was during the "prep" period when hypotension in 2 patients necessitated the administration of phenylephrine to increase diastolic blood pressure. Intubation and sternotomy produced similar increases in RPP (oxygen consumption) in these patients, but the diastolic hypotension encountered in Group N during prep theoretically could reduce myocardial blood flow to jeopardized regions of the heart. However, there was no EKG evidence of myocardial ischemia in these patients. Our conclusions are that patients on nifedipine may be safely anesthetized, but that hypotension may occur during times of lack of stimulation after induction. Hypotension is easily treated by administration of an alpha adrenergic agonist and discontinuation of the gaseous anesthetic agents.

Perioperative Uses

Calcium entry blockers are valuable new drugs in the treatment of many cardiovascular diseases. Because of the prevalence of these diseases, anesthesiologists will anesthetize many patients maintained on Ca^{++} antagonists and will wish to administer them to some patients under their care. Table 4 contains the perioperative uses of Ca^{++} entry blockers.

Table 4.

POSSIBLE PERIOPERATIVE USES OF CALCIUM CHANNEL BLOCKERS

Supraventricular Cardiac Arrhythmias
Coronary Spasm Myocardial Ischemia
Mocardial Ischemia
Cerebral Vasospasm
Hypertension
Elective Hypotension
Myocardial Protection During Cardiac Operation (Cardioplegia, Reperfusion)
Uterine Relaxation

Verapamil is useful for the treatment of supraventricular arrhythmias whereas nifedipine and verapamil are indicated in the treatment of coronary vasospasm and cerebral artery spasm. Nifedipine is probably the preferred antihypertensive and myocardial protective agent. Both can be used for uterine relaxation, perhaps nifedipine might be better in eclamptic patients. Verapamil is available for parenteral use whereas nifedipine is not. Nifedipine must be given by nasal or oral instillation since it is not available in parenteral form.

Conclusion

The advent of calcium entry blockers gives the anesthesiologist new approaches to clinical problems and they also pose new drug interaction problems. There is no good information regarding whether or not the drugs need to be discontinued for a specified interval before anesthesia, but our clinical experience with both compounds is that they may be safely continued right up to and including the morning or surgery. Both nifedipine and verapamil are potent vasodilators and must be administered with caution during anesthesia and in the perioperative period, especially in patients with impaired ventricular function and/or hypovolemia. Additionally, verapamil may produce varying degrees of A-V block and must be given very carefully in patients anesthetized with enflurane, isoflurane and halothane, in patients with A-V nodal block, or in patients maintained on beta adrenergic blocking drugs. There is little experience to guide the anesthesiologists in the perioperative use of these drugs, but their potential uses are great. The calcium channel blockers are an important addition to our formulary, with many of their uses by anesthesiologists yet to be confirmed or discovered.

REFERENCES

1. Reves JG, Kissin I, Lell WA, et al. Calcium entry blockers: uses and implications for anesthesiologists. Anesthesiology (in press).
2. McAuley BJ, Schroeder JS. The use of diltiazem hydrochloride in cardiovascular disorders. Pharmacotherapy 1982;2:121-133.
3. Fleckenstein A. Specific pharmacology of calcium in myocardium, cardiac pacemakers, and vascular smooth muscle. Annu Rev Pharmacol Toxicol 1977;17:149-166.
4. Antman EM, Stone PH, Muller JE, et al. Calcium channel blocking agents in the treatment of cardiovascular disorders. Part I: Basic and clinical electrophysiologic effects. Ann Intern Med 1980;93:875-885.
5. Henry PD. Comparative pharmacology of calcium antagonists: nifedipine, verapamil and diltiazem. Am J Cardiol 1980;46:1047-1058.
6. Stone PH, Antman EM, Muller JE, et al. Calcium channel blocking agents in the treatment of cardiovascular disorders. Part II: Hemodynamic effects and clinical applications. Ann Intern Med 1980;93:886-904.
7. Vanhoutte PM. Calcium-entry blockers and vascular smooth muscle. Circulation (Suppl I) 1982;65:I11-I19.
8. Schomerus M, Spiegelhalder B, Stieren B, et al. Physiological disposition of verapamil in man. Cardiovasc Res 1976;10:605-612.
9. Dominic JA, Bourne DWA, Tan TG, et al. The pharmacology of verapamil. III. Pharmacokinetics in normal subjects after intravenous drug administration. J Cardiovasc Pharmacol 1981;3:25-38.
10. Kates RE, Keefe DLD, Schwartz J, et al. Verapamil disposition kinetics in chronic atrial fibrillation. Clin Pharmacol Ther 1981;30:44-51.
11. Merin RG, Pask HC. The myocardial cell and it's metabolism. In: Prys-Roberts ed. The Circulation During Anesthesia. Blackwells: Oxford, 1980:3-28.
12. Komai H, Rusy BF. Effect of halothane on rested-state and potentiated-state contractions in rabbit papillary muscle: relationship to negative inotropic action. Anesth Analg (in press).
13. Price HL, Ohnishi ST. Effects of anesthetics on the heart. Fed Proc 1980;39:1575-1579.
14. Altura BM, Altura BT, Carella A, et al. Vascular smooth muscle and general anesthetics. Fed Proc 1980;39:1584-1591.
15. Blanck TJ, Thompson M: Calcium transport by cardiac sarcoplasmic reticulum: modulation of halothane action by substrate concentration and pH. Anesth Analg 1981;60:390-394.
16. Atlee JL III, Alexander SC. Halothane effects on conductivity of the AV node and his-purkinje system in the dog. Anesth Analg 1977;56:378-386.
17. Atlee JL III, Rusy BF. Atrioventricular conduction times and atrioventricular nodal conductivity during enflurane anesthesia in dogs. Anesthesiology 1977;47:498-503.
18. Atlee JL III, Rusy BF, Kreul JF, et al. Supraventricular excitability in dogs during anesthesia with halothane and enflurane. Anesthesiology 1978;49:407-413.
19. Lynch C, Vogel S, Sperelakis N. Halothane depresses cardiac slow action potentials. Anesthesiology 1980;53:S420.
20. Kapur PA, Flacke WE. Epinephrine induced arrhythmias and cardiovascular function after verapamil during halothane anesthesia in the dog. Anesthesiology 1981;55:218-225.

21. Kapur PA, Flacke WE, Olewine SK. Comparison of effects of isoflurane versus enflurane on cardiovascular and catecholamine responses to verapamil in dogs. Anesth Analg 1982;61:193-194.
22. Kates RA, Kaplan JA, Hug CC, et al: Hemodynamic interactions of verapamil and isoflurane in dogs. Anesth Analg 1982;61:194-195.
23. Brichard G, Zimmermann PE. Verapamil in cardiac dysrhythmias during anaesthesia. Br J Anaesth 1970;42:1005-1012.
24. Kapur PA, Flacke WE. Lack of correlation of verapamil plasma level with cumulative protective effects against halothane - epinephrine ventricular arrhythmias. J Cardiovasc Pharmacol 1982;4:652-657.
25. Kraynack BJ, Lawson NW, Gintautas J. Effects of verapamil on excitable membranes. Proc West Pharmacol Soc 1982;25 (in press).
26. Tosone SR, Reves JG, Kissin I, et al. Nifedipine and halothane: additive hemodynamic depression in dogs. Anesth Analg 1982;61:218-219.
27. Tosone S, Reves JG, Kissin I, et al. Hemodynamic interaction of nifedipine and halothane in dogs. Anesthesiology 1982;57:A4.

COMPARISONS BETWEEN BETA BLOCKERS AND CALCIUM ENTRY BLOCKERS

J. H. TINKER, M.D.

The Beta Blockers

In cardiology and related areas, if the decade of the 70's could be called the decade of the beta blockers, there are those who believe that the decade of the 80's will be called the decade of the calcium entry blockers.[1,2] Recently, 11 separate beta adrenergic blocking agents were licensed in Great Britain.[3] As of this writing, there are five beta adrenergic blocking agents licensed in the United States, only one of which, namely propranolol, is licensed for intravenous use in this country (see Table 1). Many of your patients will be, nowadays, taking some of these "new generation" beta blockers. An important point to make with respect to beta blockers compared to calcium entry blockers is that the beta blockers are, essentially, very similar drugs. By this I mean that if a drug is classified a beta adrenergic blocking agent, then its effect is known and predictable. It is a "negative" drug. It removes adrenergic influence on myocardium, blood vessels, and, if it crosses the blood-brain barrier, on the brain itself. Beta adrenergic blockers are not, directly, in the dosages prescribed either orally or intravenously, negative inotropic or chronotropic agents. If the administration of a beta adrenergic blocking agent reduces heart rate and/or contractility, it is via reduction of adrenergic influence. In this sense, the beta adrenergic blockers are analogous to atropine which also has no influence other than the removal of cholinergic activity, at least in reasonable doses. Thus beta adrenergic blocking agents are a) pharmacologically very similar even if they are different pharmacokinetically; b) negative drugs, i.e. they remove adrenergic influence but are not, at least in clinical dosage, direct negative inotropes or chronotropes. The clinical relevance of this is that if your patient is taking nadolol (Corgard®) preoperatively, although the compound is much longer acting than propranolol and thus would be expected to result in relatively high levels of beta adrenergic blockade throughout operation, you can be confident that the effects of the drug are not dissimilar to those of propranolol itself. Thus, although there may be numerous other beta adrenergic blocking agents marching acorss the Atlantic toward us like the broomsticks in Walt Disney's "The Sorcerer's Apprentice", we can be ready for them, secure in the knowledge that once we have understood beta adrenergic blockade, all we need do is understand which drugs are long acting and which are not. In the latter regard, the only U.S.-licensed beta blocker which is significantly longer acting than propranolol in this author's opinion, is the drug nadolol (Corgard®). Although some of the others are touted to be so, this author is unimpressed that their blood levels remain elevated significantly longer.

There is one other aspect of beta blockers which needs to be mentioned, namely beta I vs. beta II. Again, much is made of these differential effects in the literature which is attempting to induce cardiologists to prescribe one vs. the other. Propranolol, the prototype, is, of course, possessed of both beta I and the bothersome beta II blocking effects. This makes propranolo less desirable in the presence of asthma, etc. Further, propranolol beta II blocking effects may cause problems for diabetics because release of glucose from the liver in response to epinephrine is a beta II effect. This can become important if your diabetic patient was given half his or her morning dose of NPH or Lente insulin on the morning of surgery and your replacement of glucose was inadequate. Now it is 11 a.m., blood sugar is extremely low, your patient is severely hypoglycemic, and is releasing epinephrine to stimulate hepatic glucose release. If that patient was on propranolol, the hepatic beta II receptors may be at least partially blocked. Both of these two effects obviously depend on "adequate" blood levels of propranolol. We and others, measuring blood propranolol levels, have been shocked and chagrined that if the patient's propranolol was stopped at midnight, and if the patient was taking usual doses of propranolol, i.e. 160 mg/day or less, that blood levels of propranolol on entrance to the operating room, even for an 8 a.m. case, are so low as to be negligible.[4,5] Clearly, if adequate blood propranolol levels are desired, the 6 a.m. dose should be given with a small sip of water for an 8 a.m. case, and the noon dose should be given for an afternoon case.

The other four beta blockers licensed for U.S. use have a variety of different percentages of beta I vs. beta II. The reason I have downplayed the importance of this for anesthesiologists is as follows. Most of the effort in the pharmaceutical industry with respect to the beta blockers has been in the arena of reduction of side effects. By side effects I really mean beta II blockade mostly. Thus, if your preanesthetic patient is on a beta blocker which has, in that patient, successfully managed to reduce the beta II side effects, then your anesthetic will be even easier to administer. If you can manage a patient who is taking oral propranolol, then you can manage a patient who is taking any of the other beta blockers. Difficulties in anesthetic management, and requirements of reduction of volatile agent dosage, will be dependent on relative blood level of the agent, not on whether the blocker is more or less cardioselective. Table 1 delineates these agents and their rough half lives as well as beta I vs. beta II blocking properties.

Table 1. Beta blockers available in USA

Generic Name	Brand Name	Selectivity	Duration	IV Form Available
Propranolol	Inderal®	β_1,β_2	3-4 hrs half life	Yes
Metoprolol	Lopressor®	β_1	3-4 hrs half life	No
Timolol	Blocadren®	β_1,β_2	4-5 hrs half life	No
Nadolol	Corgard®	β_1,β_2	20 hrs half life	No
Atenolol	Tenormin®	β_1	6-8 hrs half life	No

The Calcium Entry Blockers

Many anesthetists, I think, were hoping that the calcium entry blockers would be as easy and pleasant to get along with as were the beta blockers. We learned early that the beta blockers should definitely not be stopped prior to anesthesia and surgery. If anything, their presence merely necessitated a reduction in volatile agent dosage or a switch to narcotic-based anesthesia. Unfortunately, and potentially dangerously, I believe that the calcium entry blockers may be more difficult to get along with during anesthesia and surgery. In addition to their individual pharmacology noted below, many internists are combining beta blockers and calcium entry blockers in patients about to undergo anesthesia and surgery. The internists' age-old philosphy of "if a little is good, a lot must be better" may have reached a "breaking point" here. It seems logical that if you depress your patient's cardiovascular system enough with drugs such as beta blockers which remove adrenergic influence, calcium blockers which directly depress inotropic state, that you will, sooner or later, reach a point at which no further depression of this patient's cardiovascular system, to any significant degree, will be tolerated. Enter the hapless anesthetist with his syringe of pentothal. Patients on both calcium entry blockers and beta blockers, if the blood levels of each are high at the time of anesthesia and surgery, may not tolerate further cardiovascular depression. What I am trying to say is that because it was logical, and has been proven valid not to stop beta blockers, it has not yet been proved that calcium entry blockers, especially if added on top of beta blockers, should also be continued, especially in high dosage, right up to and through surgery.

The main teaching point with respect to calcium entry blockers as they are compared to beta blockers is that they are all different pharmacologically. There are only two calcium entry blockers licensed for use in the United States. Verapamil, very recently licensed for oral use, is the only drug licensed for intravenous use. Nifedipine, licensed for oral use, probably will never be licensed for intravenous use because of its instability. Diltiazem, a drug fairly similar to nifedipine as near as can be estimated on the basis of preliminary drug trials, is more stable and should be available shortl for intravenous use. Thus it is fair to say that we will probably have a nifedipine-like drug available for operating room use soon.

Verapamil selectively depresses the AV node. Acute myocardial ischemia may present with development of varying degrees of AV block. Verapamil is not indicated in the treatment of this kind of myocardial ischemia. If you failed to notice that the PR interval had lengthened considerably in your patient who has just developed ST-segment depression, and you give this patient a dose of verapamil, the result may be disastrous development of complete or second degree AV block, severe low output syndrome, hypotension, inadequate coronary perfusion, and a vicious cycle leading to either myocardial infarction or death. Verapamil is indicated for the treatment of supraventricular tachydysrhythmias such as are seen in digitalis toxicity, perhaps in Wolff-Parkinson White syndrome (although this is controversial), during emergency from cardiopulmonary bypass, perhaps in rapid atrial fibrillation, and such syndromes which have, for one reason or another, generated an acute supraventricular tachydysrhythmia. It is the first and only available antidysrhythmic agent which works at or above the AV node and is thus a dramatic breakthrough. It does indeed depress myocardial oxygen consumption but because of its selective activity on the AV node, in my opinion, will not prove very useful in the treatment of acute intraoperative myocardial ischemia, because of the AV nodal effects of anesthetics and ischemia.

Nifedipine, recently studied acutely,[6] is a very different drug. Its acute usage results in humans in tachycardia instead of the bradycardia we expect from verapamil. Obviously, there are calcium channels and then there are other types of calcium channels! Nifedipine directly depresses myocardial oxygen consumption as usual and it is a potent vasodilator. Probably, at least in its acute administration, its effects in lower doses are largely those of a peripheral vasodilator. The tachycardia is thus a reflex tachycardia. If the patient is already beta-blocked as may well be the case in the presence of acute myocardial ischemia in the operating room, then nifedipine (or diltiazem) would not be likely to cause reflex tachycardia and may be useful in therapy, assuming that removal of adrenergic influence by beta blockade was not sufficient treatment. At present, because nifedipine is unavailable for intravenous usage, I do not believe that there is a calcium entry blocker available in the U.S. which should be a first-line drug for intraoperative myocardial ischemia. There are those who would advocate breaking open a capsule of nifedipine and administering the drug sublingually. This is, to say the least, an erratic route of administration for a patient who is in the throes of acute myocardial ischemia.

Many other calcium entry blockers are on the horizon, i.e. being used in Europe. Because of the incredibly expensive and complex procedures required for introduction of a new drug in the U.S., many of these will never enter our market. My major point, however, is that when a new calcium entry blocker does enter our market, not only must we become familiar with its pharmacokinetics but we need also to become familiar with it as an individual drug because the calcium entry blockers are quite different from one another, in sharp contrast to the beta blockers.

In summary, the beta blockers are negative or "take away" drugs which remove adrenergic influence but are not direct negative inotropes or chronotropes themselves, in sharp contrast to calcium entry blockers. Beta blockers are a very uniform class of drugs. If you understand the effects of beta blockade (with the nuances of beta I vs. beta II) then you understand virtually all the beta blockers. The calcium entry blockers are individual drugs, each with specific and sometimes diametrically opposed effects. For example, verapamil has selective AV nodal depressant effects and is therefore nearly always productive of a directly induced decrease in heart rate. This leads to its major use, namely the treatment of various supraventricular tachydysrhythmias. Nifedipine is a myocardial depressant and vasodilator (as is verapamil) without specific effect on the AV node. If reductions in arterial blood pressure occur acutely, then nifedipine produces reflex tachycardia. Finally, it is too early in the evolution of our knowledge of calcium entry blockers to make sweeping statements about them with respect to anesthetics. Flacke and Kapur[7] have shown in dogs that the myocardial depressant effects of verapamil are additive to those of the volatile agents, as you would expect. The combination of beta blockade and calcium entry blockade, coupled with anesthetics, has not yet been studied. It seems to me that the cardiovascular system is a bit of a waterfall, in the sense that you can only depress it so far before you get to the point wherein an additional depressant may drop the cardiac output into nonviability. We do not know enough yet to advise you as to whether to stop one or the other of the two drugs or both or neither. My own current practice is to stop neither but to induce anesthesia with extrem caution and with monitors placed awake. The decade of the 80's may be the decade of the calcium entry blockers or it could be a decade of major problems for those of us who are required to give additional myocardial depressants, namely anesthetics.

References

1. Cohn JN, Editor, Calcium entry blockers in coronary artery disease. Am Heart Assoc Monograph No. 84. Circulation 65:I1-I59, 1981
2. McGoon MD, Vlietstra RE, Holmes DR, et al: The clinical use of verapamil. Proc Mayo Clin 57:495, 1982
3. Marshall AJ: Drug therapy of hypertension and ischemic heart disease. Br J Anaesth 53:697-709, 1981
4. Sill JC, Nugent M, Moyer TP, et al: Influence of propranolol blood levels on hemodynamic response to surgical stimulation in man. Anesthesiology 57:A5, 1982
5. Sill JC, Tinker JH, Nugent M, et al: Halothane not effective in treatment of stress-induced elevation of pulmonary capillary wedge pressure. Anesthesiology 57:A60, 1982
6. Majid PA, DeJong J: Acute hemodynamic effects of nifedipine in patients with ischemic heart disease. Circulation 65:1114-1118, 1982
7. Kapur PA, Flacke WE: Epinephrine-induced arrhythmias and cardiovascular function after verapamil during halothane anesthesia in the dog. Anesthesiology 55:218-225, 1981

ASPIRATION IN OBSTETRICS: ETIOLOGY, PREVENTION AND TREATMENT

CHARLES P. GIBBS, M.D.

Aspiration of gastric contents continues to be a major cause of anesthetic related maternal mortality.[1]

I. Incidence - difficult to assess because only deaths are reported, and many of these are missed.

II. Morbidity and Mortality

   A. Mortality - 3-60%[2,3,4] and depends on type aspirate, volume of aspirate, early recognition and treatment. For example, acid aspirate produces more lung damage than non-acid aspirate, and partially digested food stuff produces even morc damage,[5,6,7]

   B. Morbidity[3]

      1. Average hospital stay - 21 days.
      2. Complications: pneumonia, lung abscess, GI hemorrhage, renal failure, pulmonary embolus, etc.
      3. Again, depends on type aspirate, early recognition and treatment.

III. Pathophysiology

   A. Large chunks produce obstruction.

   B. Non-acid liquid produces brief episodes of hypoxia without permanent histological damage.[5,6]

   C. Acid liquid ($pH < 2.5$) produces a chemical burn resulting in prolonged hypoxemia and a histological picture of hemorrhage, exudate and alveolar-capillary breakdown.[5,6,7]

D. Partially digested non-acid foodstuff produces prolonged hypoxemia and a histological picture consisting of inflammation, hemorrhage and edema.[7]

E. Partially digested acid foodstuff produces severe, prolonged hypoxemia, acidosis and hypercarbia. The histological picture is one of inflammation, hemorrhagic pulmonary edema, and septal necrosis.[7]

IV. Patient at "high risk" for aspiration.[8]

A. <u>pH < 2.5</u>.[7,9,10,11]

B. <u>Volume > 25 ml</u>,[8] but not well documented.[12,13]

V. Pregnancy predisposes to "high risk" state

A. In labor or not

1. 29% of patients <u>in labor</u> have > 25 ml of gastric contents with pH < 2.5.[8]

2. 25% of patients <u>not in labor</u> have > 25 ml of gastric contents with pH < 2.5.[8]

B. Why are pregnant patients at risk?

1. Physiology of pregnancy.

a. Increased gastrin secretion.[14]

b. Increased gastric pressure.[15]

c. Prolonged gastric emptying time during labor.[16,17]

2. Additional risks - often iatrogenic.

a. Narcotics - prolonged gastric emptying time[16,18,19] even more.

b. Pushing on uterus at time of delivery further increases intraabdominal and intragastric pressure.

c. Anesthesia

a. Decreased consciousness.

b. Paralyzed vocal cords.

c. Increased intragastric pressure secondary to succinylcholine fasciculations.[20]

VI. Signs and symptoms

A. Vomiting or regurgitation <u>may</u> be seen.

B. Wheezes <u>may</u> be heard.

C. Cyanosis <u>may</u> occur.

D. Pulmonary edema <u>may</u> occur.

E. Hypotension <u>may</u> occur.

F. X-ray - findings <u>may</u> be present, but may also be delayed, and <u>can</u> be absent.[4,21,22]

G. <u>Hypoxemia</u> - earliest and most reliable sign despite type of material and pH[5,7,23] If aspiration has occurred hypoxemia will be present. A blood gas determination is necessary to identify it, however. Therefore, if there is any suspicion of aspiration, a blood gas is indicated. If low, treatment is indicated.

VII. Treatment

A. Prevention - obviously the best.

B. Suction.

C. Supportive - may require fluids, vasopressors and/or cardiotonic drugs.

D. Antibiotics - only when indicated.

E. Steroids[24,25] - of no proven benefit physiologically and may be histologically harmful particularly following foodstuff aspiration.[26] These agents can inhibit the foreign body response and alter the normal healing process following foodstuff aspiration.[26]

F. Saline lavage - again, of little proven benefit and may serve only to disseminate aspiration material further. Moreover, the instillation of saline into the tracheobronchial tube may make the hypoxia worse.

G. Positive pressure ventilation with positive end expiratory pressure.[27] After clearing the airway, this step is the first and most important measure that can be taken. Without it, therapy has really not begun.

VIII. Prevention

A. No oral intake once labor has begun. We must convince patients not to eat before entering the hospital. For the most part, we can convert acid liquid to non-acid liquid with the use of antacids or cimetidine. Non-acid liquid is relatively benign. However, even non-acid partially digested food produces significant damage.

B. Regional anesthesia when feasible

1. Cesarean section.
2. Vaginal delivery.

C. If general anesthesia necessary:

1. Antacids

a. Antacids originally suggested by Taylor and Pryse-Davies to elevate pH of stomach contents.[28]

b. Roberts and Shirley popularized in U.S.[8]

c. Antacids did elevate pH, but did not reduce mortality.[8,29,30,31]

d. Particulate antacids found to be physiologically and histologically damaging.[5,32]

e. A clear, non-particulate antacids such as 0.3 M Na Citrate is a safe and effective alternative.[33,34,35]

1) However, it is not commercially available and, therefore, must be prepared by hospital pharmacy - a nuisance.

2) Formula

Sodium citrate	88.2 g
Simple syrup	100.0 ml
Mint flavor	1.0 ml
H_2O	1000.0 ml

f. $NaHCO_3$, orally administered intravenous preparation (20 ml) is also effective[36] and is readily available in all hospitals and on all wards. It is not very palatable, however.

g. Bicitra is a commercially available antacid, appears safe and should be effective.[37]

2. Following administration of antacids, rotate patient back and forth to ensure adequate mixing.[38]
3. Cimetidine[39]

   a. 300 mg hs + 300 mg IM morning before surgery is effective and has no adverse effects on newborn.

   b. 300 mg IV? - may produce hypotension.
4. Glycopyrrolate decreases gastric acidity,[41] but also decreases esophageal sphincter tone.[42]
5. Metoclopramide decreases gastric emptying time [43] and <u>increases</u> esophageal sphincter tone.[44]
6. Nasogastric tube - doubtful value.[45]
7. Emetics - doubtful value.[45]
8. Precurarization - to decrease rise in intragastric pressure secondary to succinylcholine,[20] but is it necessary? The rise in intragastric pressure is paralled by a rise in pressure above the gastroesophageal sphincter.[46] Also, muscle relaxation may be quicker and more profound without precurarization and, therefore intubation easier.
9. Rapid sequence induction or awake intubation.

10. Head up.
11. Cricoid pressure - simple and very effective if properly applied - very important.[1,45,46,47] Person applying it must know when and how, and must <u>never</u> release pressure until tube in place.
12. Cuffed endotracheal tube.
13. Tube definitely in place before surgery begins. If intubation proves difficult or impossible, and the operation has not begun, the patient can be allowed to awaken and the entire situation reassessed. However, if the incision is already made, the option of allowing the patient to awaken is eliminated.
14. Awake extubation, because the threat of aspiration is present at extubation as well as at intubation.

REFERENCES

1. Tomkinson J, Turnbull A, Robson, G, et al: Report on Confidential Enquiries into Maternal Deaths in England and Wales 1973-1975. Her Majesty's Stationery Office, 1979.
2. Mendelson CL: The aspiration of stomach contents into the lungs during obstetric anesthesia. Am J Obstet Gynecol 52:191, 1946.
3. Arms RA, Dines DE, Tinstman TC: Aspiration pneumonia. Chest 65:136, 1974.
4. Cameron JL, Mitchell WH, Zuidema GD: Aspiration pneumonia. Clinical outcome following documented aspiration. Arch Surg 106:49, 1973.
5. Gibbs CP, Schwartz DJ, Wynne JW, et al: Antacid pulmonary aspiration in the dog. Anesthesiology 51:380, 1979.
6. Teabeaut JR II: Aspiration of gastric contents. An experimental study. Am J Pathol 28:51, 1952.
7. Schwartz DJ, Wynne JW, Gibbs CP, et al: The pulmonary consequences of aspiration of gastric contents at pH values greater than 2.5. Amer Rev Respir Dis 121:119, 1980.

8. Roberts RB, Shirley MA: The obstetrician's role in reducing the risk of aspiration pneumonitis. With particular reference to the use of oral antacids. Am J Obstet Gynecol 124:611, 1976.
9. Bannister WK, Sattilaro AJ: Vomiting and aspiration during anesthesia. Anesthesiology 23:251, 1962.
10. Vandam LD: Aspiration of gastric contents in the operative period. N Engl J Med 273:1206, 1965.
11. Awe WC, Fletcher WS, Jacob SW: The pathophysiology of aspiration pneumonitis. Surgery 60:232, 1966.
12. Exarhos ND, Logan WD, Abbott OA, et al: The importance of pH and volume in tracheobronchial aspiration. Dis Chest 47:167, 1965.
13. Modell JH, Gibbs CP, Kuck EJ, et al: Aspiration: Combined effects of pH and volume. Abstracts of Scientific Papers. S.O.A.P. Meeting, June 2-6, 1982, p 39.
14. Attia RR, Ebeid AM, Fischer JE, et al: Maternal fetal and placental gastrin concentrations. Anaesthesia 37:18, 1982.
15. O'Mullane EJ: Vomiting and regurgitation during anesthesia. Lancet 1:1209, 1954.
16. LaSalvia LA, Steffen EA: Delayed gastric emptying time in labor. Am J Obstet Gynecol 59:1075, 1950.
17. Davison JS, Davison MC, Hay DM: Gastric emptying time in late pregnancy and labour. J Obstet Gynaecol Brit Common 77:37, 1970.
18. Holdsworth JD: Relationship between stomach contents and analgesia in labour. Brit J Anaesth 50:1145, 1978.
19. Nimmo WS, Wilson J, Prescott LF: Narcotic analgesics and delayed gastric emptying during labour. Lancet 1:890, 1975.
20. Miller RD, Way WL: Inhibition of succinylcholine-induced increased intragastric pressure by nondepolarizing muscle relaxants and lidocaine. Anesthesiology 34:185, 1971.
21. Cameron JL, Anderson RP, Zuidema GD: Aspiration pneumonia. A clinical and experimental review. J Surg Res 7:44, 1967.
22. Landay MJ, Christensen EE, Bynum LJ: Pulmonary manifestations of acute aspiration of gastric contents. Am J Roentgenol 131:587, 1978.
23. Wynne JW, Hood CI: Hypoxemia in the first hour after aspiration. Chest 78:3, 1980.
24. Downs JB, Chapman RL, Modell JH, et al: An evaluation of steroid therapy in aspiration pneumonitis. Anesthesiology 40:129, 1974.
25. Wynne JW, DeMarco FJ, Hood CI: Physiological effects of corticosteroids in foodstuff aspiration. Arch Surg 116:46, 1981.
26. Wynne JW, Reynolds JC, Hood CI, et al: Steroid therapy for pneumonitis induced in rabbits by aspiration of foodstuff. Anesthesiology 51:11, 1979.
27. Chapman RL, Downs JB, Modell JH, et al: The ineffectiveness of steroid therapy in treating

aspiration of hydrochloric acid. Arch Surg 108:858, 1974.
28. Taylor G, Pryse-Davies J: The prophylactic use of antacids in the prevention of the acid-pulmonary-aspiration syndrome (Mendelson's syndrome). Lancet, February 5, 1966, p 288.
29. Bond VK, Stoelting RK, Gupta CD: Pulmonary aspiration syndrome after inhalation of gastric fluid containing antacids. Anesthesiology 51:452, 1979.
30. Scott DB: Mendelson's syndrome. (Editorial) Brit J Anaesth 50:81, 1978.
31. Taylor G: Acid pulmonary aspiration syndrome after antacids: A case report. Brit J Anaesth 47:615, 1975.
32. Gibbs CP, Kuck EJ, Hood CI, et al: Antacid plus foodstuff aspiration in the dog. Anesthesiology 53:S307, 1980.
33. Lahiri SK, Thomas TA, Hodgson RMH: Single-dose antacid therapy for the prevention of Mendelson's syndrome. Brit J Anaesth 45:1143, 1973.
34. Hester JB, Heath ML: Pulmonary acid aspiration syndrome: Should prophylaxis be routine? Brit J Anaesth 49:595, 1977.
35. Gibbs CP, Spohr L, Schmidt D: The effectiveness of sodium citrate as an antacid. Anesthesiology 57:0046, 1982.
36. Lim HS, Tan PL: Sodium bicarbonate, injection, U.S.P. as an oral antacid for emergency cesarean section patients. Anesthesiology 55(3):A339, 1981.
37. Eyler SW, Cullen BF, Murphy ME, et al: Antacid aspiration in rabbits: A comparison of mylanta and bicitra. Anesth Analg 61:288, 1982.
38. Holdsworth JD, Johnson K, Mascall G, et al: Mixing of antacids with stomch contents. Another approach to the prevention of the acid aspiration (Mendelson's) syndrome. Anaesthesia 35:641, 1980.
39. Manchikanti L, Kraus JW, Edds SP: Cimetidine and related drugs in anesthesia. Anesth Analg 61(7):595, 1982.
40. Shaw RG, Mashford ML, Desmond PV: Cardiac arrest after intravenous injection of cimetidine. Med J Aust 2:629, 1980.
41. Baraka A, Saab M, Salem MR, et al: Control of gastric acidity by glycopyrrolate premedication in the parturient. Anesth Analg 56:642, 1977.
42. Brock-Utne JG, Welman RS, Dimopoulos GE, et al: The effect of glycopyrrolate (Robinul) on the lower oesophageal sphincter. Canad Anaesth Soc J 25:144, 1978.
43. Howard FA, Sharp DS: Effect of metoclopramide on gastric emptying during labour. Brit Med J, 1:446, 1973.
44. Laitinen S, Mokka REM, Valanne JVI, et al: Anaesthesia induction and lower oesophageal sphincter pressure. Acta Anaesth Scand 22:16, 1978.
45. Holdsworth JD, Furness RMB, Roulston RG: A comparison

of apomorphine and stomach tubes for emptying the stomach before general anaesthesia in obstetrics. Brit J Anaesth 45:526, 1974.

46. Smith G, Dalling R, William TIR: Gastro-oesophageal pressure gradient changes produced by induction of anaesthesia and suxamethonium. Brit J Anaesth 50:1137, 1978.
47. Salem MR, Wong AY, Fizzotti GF: Efficacy of cricoid pressure in preventing aspiration of gastric contents in paediatric patients. Brit J Anaesth 44:401, 1972.
48. Sellick BA: Cricoid pressure to control regurgitation of stomach contents during induction of anaesthesia. Lancet II:404, 1961.

NEW DEVELOPMENTS IN VASODILATOR THERAPY

J. H. TINKER, M.D.

INTRODUCTION

With the demonstration by Franciosa et al[1] in 1973 that patients who were in severe congestive failure could sometimes (with great variability) be dramatically helped to large increases in cardiac output by afterload reduction with nitroprusside; the idea of utilizing afterload reduction as therapy "caught on" rapidly after generations of trying to "get the blood pressure up". The idea of "reducing the workload" of the heart by decreasing vascular resistance was one whose time had come. The reasons it didn't always work are complex. Often, physicians ignored reflex effects of their reductions in vascular resistance. The degree of intactness of said reflexes depends on prior drug therapy, inherent cardiac reserve, and in our case, the presence of myocardially depressant anesthetics and their adjuvants such as beta blocker

Into this milieu jumped the usual "advocates". There were those who advocated nitroprusside, others advocated nitroglycerin. Still others stuck to ganglionic blocking agents of the past such as trimethaphan. Another group thought that the direct peripheral vasodilating actions of halothane, ethrane, and forane, coupled with their anesthetizing properties, was simplest and therefore made the most sense. Recently, with the calcium entry blockers came the realization that these drugs, negative inotropes for vascular smooth muscle, are often primarily peripheral vasodilators. Can we, then, decide when to use peripheral vasodilation as a form of therapy and are there, now, solid indications as to which type to use?

Indications for Vasodilator Therapy

Intraoperative myocardial ischemia, evidenced by ST-segment depression, has been thought in the past to be a prime indication for nitroglycerin therapy More recently, it has been recognized that if there is concomitant tachycardia, the latter should be treated first (with beta blockers) before or during vasodilator therapy. Intraoperative myocardial ischemia *per se* is not an indication for vasodilator therapy unless that ischemia is thought due to circulatory hyperdynamism. Hyperdynamism can be due to high afterload, high heart rate, or both. Other perioperative uses for vasodilator therapy usually include hypertension syndromes of various sorts. There is no question that severe intra- and postoperative hypertension occurs during abdominal and thoracic aortic surgery, after aortic valve replacement, and often after coronary artery bypass. Perhaps disturbances of afferent reflex pathways by traumatizing the aorta itself are responsible for some of this hypertension. Levels of systolic arterial pressure seen in these patients are often alarmingly high. Clearly vasodilator therapy is called for in such circumstances and we would administer the vasodilator first, in this case but we would be very aware of, and worried about, the possibility of reflex tachycardia. We would add beta blocker therapy to our vasodilator should that occur. Some would say that if you measure cardiac output and you find a peripheral vascular resistance of, say, 1800 dynes cm^{-5} sec^{-1} that you should administer a vasodilator to lower that number to, say 1200. This is nonsense in the sense that you are treating an isolated number. In the first place, because you are multiplying by 80 in order to get into the CGS units, you are multiplying all your errors by 80! There is a range of normality in peripheral vascular resistance, especially in the above units, which is very wide. If your patient's heart rate is relatively low, the arterial pressure is reasonable, if hemodynamics have been stable for some time and if urinary output is progressing reasonably, we would not treat this isolated number. If on the other hand, we had a low output situation with a high peripheral vascular resistance, then resistance can and should be used to gauge vasodilator therapy efficacy.

Which Vasodilator to Use

Chiariello et al[2] in 1976 compared nitroprusside to nitroglycerin in patients who had suffered acute myocardial infarctions. They found, at comparable preload reductions, ECG evidence of improvement during nitroglycerin therapy vs. deterioration during nitroprusside. They conducted animal experiments with radioactive microspheres and concluded that, somehow, nitroprusside seemed to be diverting blood away from the ischemic areas whereas nitroglycerin was adding blood to same. Nitroglycerin was not licensed for intravenous use, nor commercially available, until 1981. Despite this, numerous papers have advocated its use instead of nitroprusside as a vasodilator. Nitroglycerin is, therefore, the newest vasodilator on the market even though it has been used for many years in many centers. We will discuss its pharmaceutical and pharmacological nuances below. In contrast to Chiariello et al,[2] Kerber et al,[3] in dogs, could not demonstrate any differences between nitroprusside and nitroglycerin during acute experimental myocardial ischemia, in regional flow, endocardial/epicardial perfusion ratios, or in ischemia-induced resultant depression of regional function. More recently, nitroprusside and nitroglycerin were compared in the treatment of severe postoperative hypertension.[4] Many have thought that severe arterial hypertension such as occurs after aortic valve surgery demanded the use of nitroprusside because of its more effective arteriolar vasodilation properties. This recent report[4] concluded that nitroglycerin could be safely and effectively used, avoiding nitroprusside-induced cyanide toxicity, etc. and was therefore the drug of choice even for this therapy. Clearly, nitroglycerin is not only a venodilator but also an effective arteriolar dilator in many patients.

In our practice, we find ourselves using nitroglycerin when myocardial ischemia is related to the diagnosis or is thought to be imminent. We still prefer nitroprusside in many circumstances of severe arterial hypertension. One of the commonest of these occurs during cardiopulmonary bypass with time. Whether due to renin-angiotensin activation, thromboxane release, or catecholamine stimulation, arterial pressure often inexorably climbs during hypothermic cardiopulmonary bypass at constant flow. We find nitroglycerin often ineffective in reducing this pressure and continue to utilize nitroprusside. We often also use nitroprusside in treating severe postoperative hypertensive syndromes, being careful not to exceed 8 µg/kg/min because of cyanide toxicity. Addition of beta blockade and/or calcium entry blockers will greatly reduce the dosage of nitroprusside required.

Nitroglycerin - Pharmacy and Pharmacology

We seldom consider very much about the pharmacy of the drugs we use. Nitroglycerin availability was long delayed not because of pharmacology but because of pharmacy. The compound is an oily, volatile and extremely unstable substance. It adheres to glass, but especially plastics, having the ability to pass readily through many common plastics, including that of the commonly-used intravenous fluid bags and tubing. To add to its compounding problems, the substance is not very miscible in water and may separate in aqueous solution thus making dosage unreliable. The currently available intravenous preparations utilize compounding with 10% ethanol in order to minimize the miscibility problem. The pharmaceutical companies advocate administration of nitroglycerin via specially formulated heavy plastic tubing. Company literature indicates that up to 85% of the agent could be lost on passage to the patient, depending on dosage rate. It is important to remember that the pharmaceutical company has a financial stake in this number. If they can, rightly or wrongly, convince us that the drug is so unstable as to be impossible or unsafe to administer using our routine sets, then they can sell us the "special" drip sets. This author remains unconvinced that the compound is quite that difficult to administer. Nonetheless, it is fair to say that pharmaceutics are very important with respect to intravenous nitroglycerin.

The pharmacology of nitroglycerin is little in doubt. The drug is a vasodilator, but primarily a venodilator. You can expect a reasonable reduction in preload before you get severe arterial hypotension, especially if venodilation is possible. In many patients with severe chronic congestive failure, their veins are maximally dilated. Nitroglycerin is not likely to have significant beneficial preload-reducing effect. On the other hand, the usual surgical patient with reasonable myocardial function will achieve preload reduction on nitroglycerin. Unfortunately, the preload-reducing dose is not that much smaller than the arteriolar dilating dose (and in many patients hypotension may result before achievement of desired preload reduction). It is said by some that reflex tachycardia is less of a problem with nitroglycerin than nitroprusside. In fact, reflex tachycardia depends on the degree to which arterial pressure is reduced, assuming no concomitant interferences such as anesthesia, etc. Thus, if a desired preload-reducing effect occurs at less of a decrease in arterial pressure with nitroglycerin, then there will be less reflex tachycardia. Many of the literature comparisons of the two drugs utilized the same reductions in arterial pressure. Since nitroprusside is more of a generalized vasodilator, comparisons of nitroglycerin vs. nitroprusside at the same reductions in mean arterial pressure may not be entirely valid.

Nitroprusside, of course, has cyanide toxicity liability, especially as dosages get near or in excess of 8 µg/kg/min. Nitroglycerin is said by many to have no toxicity. It should be borne in mind that nitroprusside was thought to have no toxicity until 1975.[5] We may find significant liabilities to nitroglycerin, although none have been reported to date. Nitroglycerin can cause methemoglobinemia, but the clinical importance of that remains to be delineated.

With respect to nitroglycerin, although it may be reasonable to start at 1 µg/kg/min, we find the dosage required by each patient to vary considerably. Since no specific toxicity has been yet reported for nitroglycerin, we feel that titration to desired preload reduction and/or arterial pressure can be accomplished almost without regard to administered dosage.

The Calcium Channel Blockers as Vasodilators

A recent report on the hemodynamic effects of acutely administered nifedipine indicates clearly that, in reasonable doses, the major effect of this drug is that of a vasodilator.[6] Thus, patients taking oral nifedipine can be expected to be relatively "full" with respect to their vascular systems. Although this study demonstrated reflex tachycardia during the acute phase, we would expect that chronic oral nifedipine therapy would result in assumption of sufficient vascular volume so to minimize concomitant tachycardia. Verapam is not the drug of choice for use as a vasodilator because of its AV nodal selectivity.[7]

Other Vasodilators of Interest to Anesthesiologists

Numerous other vasodilators such as hydralazine, diazoxide, minoxidil, prazosin, are used by clinicians in the treatment of various hypertensive syndromes. None of these have "caught on" for intraoperative use, primarily because of long onset times coupled with variable lengths of action. None of these drugs are controllable on a minute-to-minute basis which seems to be desirable for us during anesthesia and surgery. An antihypertensive of special concern to anesthesiologists is the centrally-acting alpha adrenergic agent clonidine.[8] This drug, when it is withdrawn acutely by making the patient NPO, and when sufficient sympathetic stimulation exists such as surgical incision, can result in severe rebound hypertension. Said hypertension must be treated with a potent vasodilator, usually nitroprusside. As of this writing, intravenous clonidine is not available in the United States and so patients taking clonidine should either be switched several weeks to some other antihypertensive or left on their oral clonidine as near to surgery as possible. The anesthetist should be prepared for sudden severe episodes of hypertension during the operation itself.

References

1. Franciosa JA, Guiha NH, Limas CJ, et al: Improved left ventricular function during nitroprusside infusion in acute myocardial infarction. Lancet 1:650-654, 1972
2. Chiariello M, Gold HK, Leinbach RC, et al: Comparison between the effects of nitroprusside and nitroglycerin on ischemic injury during acute myocardiac infarction. Circulation 54:766, 1976
3. Kerber RE, Martins JB, Marcus ML: Effect of acute ischemia, nitroglycerin and nitroprusside on regional myocardial thickening, stress and perfusion. Circulation 60:121-129, 1979

4. Flaherty JT, Magee PA, Gardner TL, et al: Comparison of intravenous nitroglycerin and sodium nitroprusside for treatment of acute hypertension developing after coronary artery bypass surgery. Circulation 65:1072-1077, 1982
5. Tinker JH, Michenfelder JD: Sodium nitroprusside: pharmacology, toxicology, and therapeutics. Anesthesiology 45:340-354, 1976
6. Majid PA, DeJong J: Acute hemodynamic effects of nifedipine in patients with ischemic heart disease. Circulation 65:1114-1118, 1982
7. McGoon MD, Vlietstra RE, Holmes DR et al: The clinical use of verapamil. Proc Mayo Clin 57:495, 1982
8. Tinker JH: Perioperative hypertension. Chapter In: Clinical Pharmacology, Kaplan J, Editor, In press

ELECTROSTIMULATION AS AN ADJUNCT TO ANESTHESIA

T. H. STANLEY

A number of years ago there was great interest in electrical anesthesia.[1] Numerous laboratories throughout this country and the world began experimenting with a variety of anesthetic currents, wave forms, frequencies, etc., with some limited success in animals. Application in man, however, was usually associated with numerous serious complications, including contractures, burns, headache, pain at the area of stimulation, convulsions and death.[1] As a result of these experiences, most investigators throughout the world gave up the idea of ever producing either analgesia or anesthesia with electricity. However, a small group headquartered in France continued experiments and after some years of evaluating a variety of currents, frequencies, amplitudes, and wave forms developed a form of electrical stimulation which has most recently been called Transcutaneous Cranial Electrical Stimulation (TCES).[2,3]

It is interesting that as the work with TCES was being done in Paris, Transcutaneous Electrical Stimulation (TENS) simultaneously evolved as a clinical tool and is currently being used today to successfully treat some patients with chronic pain.[4,5] The TENS units are also being used by some investigators and clinicians to treat acute post-operative pain.[6,7]

Recent experiments in Paris have demonstrated that TCES significantly increases the potency of nitrous oxide to painful stimulation.[2] It also seems to be effective in increasing the amnesic properties of nitrous oxide as well as producing analgesia at the site of stimulation following recovery from nitrous oxide. TCES does not appear to alter circulatory and respiratory dynamics either prior to, during, or after exposure to nitrous oxide. In another series of experiments it was demonstrated that TCES is effective in reducing narcotic requirements during anesthesia with droperidol, diazepam, and pancuronium.[3] Indeed, the fentanyl requirements utilized in these patients were reduced by approximately 33%.

Recent data have indicated that electric current applied to the cranium is most analgesic when a low frequency component is part of that stimulation, 100 cycles per second or less. (Limoge A, unpublished data) However, low frequency currents capable of producing profound analgesia, also often inflict contractures, burn, and discomfort. On the other hand, very high frequencies, 167 kh, provide the advantage of not being painful to patients, indeed often not being felt by patients. In addition, high frequency currents are more capable of penetrating through the natural resistence of the skin. Unfortunately high frequencies result in less analgesia. For the above reasons, it is necessary, for optimal safety and analgesia, to mix low and high frequency currents.

The current used in the most recent TCES experiments is a mixture of low and high frequency. The current is on for 3 milliseconds and it is off for 10 milliseconds. While the current is on, the frequency is 167 kh. Another mode changes the on/off pattern to 4 milliseconds on and 8 milliseconds off and still a third mode has current on for 3 milliseconds and then off for 7 milliseconds. Recent data (Limoge A, unpublished observations) indicate that analgesia occurs with currents of 150 milliamperes or above. Currents less than this amplitude produce little analgesia with current TCES electrodes and stimulating frequencies.

The wave form of the current is complex. It is a non-sinusoidal biphasic, non-square wave pattern. Generally the peak to peak intensity ranges between 250 to 300 milliamps, depending upon patients' skin resistance. The current is delivered to the patient's cranial skin via 3 silver (paste-on) electrodes of 13.3 mm^2 area. The electrodes are applied between the eyebrows and one each over or slightly posterior to each mastoid process depending upon the patient's natural hairline.

The exact mechanism by which TCES produces analgesia is unknown at this time. Experiments are currently ongoing which hope to determine whether the current is able to increase plasma levels of beta-endorphine or any of the other endogenously produced central peptides which have been associated with analgesia.

It is clear from the most recent investigations and other unpublished observations in unanesthetized volunteers that TCES provides analgesia but not anesthesia. That TCES or any other form of TENS provides advantages when used during anesthesia has not yet been documented. Theoretically, it should be possible to use lower concentrations of inhalation anesthetics and lower doses of narcotics and other intravenous supplements when using TCES. As mentioned above, the most recent studies have documented that this is, in fact, true. As a result, major organ system alterations and functions should be less during anesthesia and post-operative recovery faster. Recovery may also be associated with residual non-chemical produced post-operative analgesia.[2] These possible advantages of TCES, if proven true in subsequent studies, could certainly alter both the research and clinical directions of anesthesiology.

REFERENCES

1. Limoge A, Debois C, Coeytaux R, et al: Electrotherapeutic sleep and electroanesthesia. Paris: Masson, 1978
2. Stanley TH, Cazaloa JA, Limoge A, et al: Transcutaneous cranial electrical stimulation increases the potency of nitrous oxide in humans. Anesthesiology (In Press)
3. Stanley TH, Cazaloa JA, Atinault A, et al: Transcutaneous cranial electrical stimulation decreases narcotic requirements during neurolept anesthesia and operation in man. Anesth Analg (In Press)
4. Long DM, Hagfors N: Electrical stimulation in the nervous system: the current status of electrical stimulation in the nervous system for the relief of pain. Pain 1:109-123, 1975

5. Thorsteinson G, Stonnington HH, Stillwell G, et al: Transcutaneous electrical stimulation: a double-blind trial of its efficacy for pain. Arch Phys Med Rehabil 58:8-13, 1977
6. Tyler E, Caldwell C, Ghia JN: Transcutaneous electrical nerve stimulation: an alternative approach to the management of postoperative pain. Anesth Analg 61:449-456, 1981
7. Ali J, Yaffe CS, Serrette C: The effects of transcutaneous electric nerve stimulation on postoperative pain and pulmonary function. Surgery 89:507-512, 1981

NEW MUSCLE RELAXANTS

JOHN J. SAVARESE, M.D.

It is widely recognized that presently available nondepolarizing relaxants may be improved in two ways: (1) by shortening their duration of effect· and (2) by eliminating their cardiovascular side effects.

Three hypothetical relaxants which might be of use to anesthetists were described seven years ago (1) (Figure 1). These were (1) a short-acting nondeporizing relaxant with onset of 1-2 minutes from injection to complete block of the adductor pollicis twitch response, and total duration of 10-20 minutes to full (90-95%) recovery (Figure 1A)· such a drug, if it also produced little or no side effects, would constitute the "ideal" relaxant. Two other hypothetical materials were also proposed as potentially clinically useful: an intermediate-duration drug without cumulative effect, and a long-acting drug with no side effects (Figure 1B and C).

Now, all three hypothetical materials are close to reality.

The "B-type" intermediate-duration, noncumulative drugs are closest to routine clinical use. In the past two years, extensive clinical trials of two promising new materials, BW 33A (atracurium) and ORG NC45 (vecuronium) have been in progress in several countries (2-5). The two new relaxants are both nondepolarizers which can be given in relatively large dosage to permit tracheal intubation within 2-3 minutes yet spontaneous recovery of the twitch response begins within approximately 30 minutes and is complete within approximately 60-90 minutes. Antagonism by anticholinesterases of residual block secondary to atracurium or vecuronium is possible within roughly 30 minutes after dosage employed for tracheal intubation. Both new drugs have relatively little side effects. In fact, vecuronium shows less cardiovascular effect than any other relaxant (2) whereas atracurium shows only a slight hypotensive effect at very high dosage, probably due to a weak histamine-releasing property which is less than that of metocurine (5,6). Atracurium, therefore, probably ranks second in terms of lack of cardiovascular effect.

Both new relaxants undergo relatively unique forms of degradation or elimination: atracurium undergoes Hofmann Elimination, a pH and temperature-sensitive degradation of the quaternary group. This mechanism is fully described in Figure 2. Vecuronium undergoes a high degree of biliary clearance of the unchanged parent molecule as well as renal clearance. The drug essentially has two routes of elimination - the kidney and the liver (7,8). The liver may possibly be the more important route (8). Comparative kinetic data for vecuronium and pancuronium in patients in renal failure are presented in Table 1. The comparative biliary elimination of vecuronium and pancuronium in rats (8) is presented in Table 2. The relatively high rate of clearance of vecuronium in bile and urine and the spontaneous breakdown (Hofmann Elimination) of atracurium contribute to a relative lack of cumulative effect in both drugs. In fact, probably because it breaks down spontaneously, atracurium shows the least cumulative property of any known nondepolarizing relaxant.

For the above reasons, both atracurium and vecuronium will be indicated in patients in renal failure, as suggested by preliminary data for both drugs. Although there is as yet no published data to support the following supposition, it might be expected that atracurium might also be indicated in patients with severe hepatobiliary disease. Because its primary route of elimination is apparently via the liver, hard data are also needed to define the elimination kinetics of vecuronium in this patient subgroup.

Because vecuronium and atracurium probably rank first and second among nondepolarizing relaxants with respect to lack of cardiovascular effect, they will also be indicated in patients with severe cardiovascular disease.

When atracurium and vecuronium become available for use (possibly in 1983), the two new relaxants will undoubtedly improve our practice pattern with respect to the provision of clinical relaxation. Where did the new drugs come from? To fully understand the impact of the two new drugs and to appreciate some of the basic scientific efforts involved in their production, it is worthwhile to describe the history of their development.

Atracurium is a bis-benzylisoquinolinium (Fig 2). As such, it is therefore a distant derivative of d-tubocurarine and its roots can be traced all the way back to the amazonian jungle vine, chondodendron tomentosum from extracts of which the indians of the amazon synthesized a paralytic arrow poison which was the original natural source of d-tubocurarine. Many isoquinolinium derivatives of d-tubocurarine have been synthesized but none (except the trimethylated semisynthetic derivative metocurine) have been acceptable for clinical use. Adaptation of benzylisoquinolinium compounds to spontaneous degradation (Hofmann Elimination) was initially described by Stenlake (9) and by Martin-Smith (10) as a route to the production of shorter-acting nondepolarizing relaxants. The impetus behind its synthesis was, therefore, the desire to obtain shorter duration of action. The developers succeeded in this regard, since atracurium has only approximately 1/3 the duration of effect of d-tubocurarine. An added bonus, which was not originally anticipated, is the fact that atracurium's cardiovascular effect is minimal (4,5).

Vecuronium (ORG NC45), Figure 3) is simply pancuronium demethylated at the 2-piperidino substitution. The history of vecuronium, and of all steroidal relaxants, interestingly enough, can also be traced back to a paralytic poison prepared by the natives of the Belgian Congo from a plant source (malouetia bequaertiana). The active principle of this plant extract is malouetine (Figure 4), a naturally occurring bisquaternary steroidal molecule. The discovery of this substance in 1960 by a group of French investigators (11) led to the synthesis of literally thousands of bisquarternary steroidal substances in quest of a clinically useful material (12). The first (and still the only clinically successful steriodal relaxant) was pancuronium, first described by Hewitt and Savage in 1964-65 (13, 13A). The brilliant chemical reasoning which sets pancuronium apart from all other steroidal relaxants is the introduction of two acetylcholine-like fragments into positions 2-3 and 16-17 in the steroidal nucleus. Later studies showed that pancuronium, although an extraordinarily potent neuromuscular blocking agent free of any hypotensive property due to either histamine release or blockade of autonomic ganglia, did often produce an increase in heart rate and arterial pressure mainly due to a vagolytic effect. These observations prompted further studies of the pancuronium series (14,15) where an important basic observation was made: the vagolytic property was mainly due to the acetylcholine-like substitution in the 2-3 position, whereas neuromuscular blocking potency is mainly attributable to the 16-17 substitution (14,15). A basic reason behind this may be the stereochemistry of the substituting groups: both piperidino substitutions are in the β position. On the other hand, the 3 and 16-acetoxy substitutions are α and β to the steroid system.

Several analogues of pancuronium were identified (15) which showed considerably less vagolytic property than pancuronium. ORG NC45 (vecuronium) emerged from the series and was chosen for development because the separation of its vagolytic property from its neuromuscular blocking action was the greatest in the series; furthermore, its duration of action in animals was considerably shorter than pancuronium.[15]

Atracurium and vecuronium do show desirable pharmacological properties and should be well accepted by anesthesiologists. They have few disadvantages, but do they fit the definition of "ideal" relaxants? In my opinion, probably not, for the following reasons: (1) relatively slow onset to abolition of twitch at fully paralyzing dosage (atracurium 0.5 mg/kg and vecuronium 0.1 mg/kg) require 4 to 5 minutes and intubation after thiopental induction cannot be smoothly accomplished until 2½ to 3 minutes after administration of the relaxant. The above times may be slightly faster than for d-tubocurarine and pancuronium, but a major difference in onset is not present. On the other hand, dosage of both drugs can be increased to provide faster onset, but then one is dealing with a patient who is fully paralyzed for 45-60 minutes before recovery begins. Whether either of the 2 drugs will replace succinylcholine for routine intubations is questionable. In situations where succinylcholine is contraindicated, however,(e.g. burned patients, paraplegics) atracurium and vecuronium will be better substitutes for intubation than presently available nondepolarizers: (2) Pharmaceutical preparation: at the present time, atracurium is supplied as a solution which requires refrigeration for storage: vecuronium is supplied as a powder with special citrated buffer to be diluted for solution before use. These preparations do offer minor inconveniences; (3) relatively slow recovery: after administration for 2 hours or more, spontaneous recovery from vecuronium block (from 95% block to 95% twitch recovery) requires 45 minutes or more because of its slight cumulative effect. Atracurium, since its cumulative effect is virtually nil, is somewhat better (30-45 minutes). Neither drug, however, allows recovery to proceed rapidly enough to eliminate the need to reverse residual block with anticholinesterase agents after most routine operations.

For the above reasons, relaxant research is continuing. Specifically, several groups are actively seeking a short-acting nondepolarizer (Drug A in Figure 1). In my opinion, a nondepolarizing relaxant which allows intubation within less than 2 minutes and full spontaneous recovery within less than ½ hour is still needed. Intermediate-duration drugs (B in Figure 1) which are stable in solution at room temperature would also offer some advantage. Finally, a long acting drug (C in Figure 1) would appear useful for long operations and for intensive care situations.

Note that any new relaxant drug, in order to gain clinical acceptance in the future, will probably have to show little or no cardiovascular effect. Vecuronium especially, and atracurium to a certain extent as well, have set new standards in this regard.

REFERENCES

1. Savarese, JJ, Kitz, RJ: Does clinical anesthesia need new neuromuscular blocking agents? Anesthesiology 42:236-239, 1975.
2. Fahey, MR., Morris, RB, Miller, RD et al: Clinical pharmacology of ORG NC45 (Norcuron TM): A new nondepolarizing relaxant. Anesthesiology 55:6-11, 1981.
3. Agoston, S, Salt, P, Newton, D et al: The neuromuscular blocking action of ORG NC45, a new pancuronium derivative, in anaesthetized patients. Br J Anaesth 52:535-539, 1980.
4. Payne, JP, Hughes, R: The evaluation of atracurium in anaesthetized man. Br J Anaesth 53:45-54, 1981.
5. Basta, SJ, Savarese, JJ, Ali, HH et al: Comparative histamine-releasing potencies of atracurium bestkate (BW 33A), metocurine and d-tubocurarine. Abstracts of Scientific Papers, ASA Meeting, 1982, Las Vegas.
6. Basta, SJ, Ali, HH, Savarese, JJ et al: Clinical pharmacology of atracurium besylate (BW 33A): a new nondepolarizing muscle relaxant. Anesth Analg (1982) In Press.
7. Fahey, MR, Morris, RB, Miller, RD, Nguyen, TL, Upton, RA et al: Pharmacokinetics of ORG NC45 (Norcuron) in patients with and without renal failure. Br J Anaesth 53:1049-1053, 1981.
8. Upton, RA, Nguyen, TL, Miller, RD, Castagnoli, N: Renal and biliary elimination of vecuronium (ORG NC45) and pancuronium in rats. Anesth Analg 61:313-316, 1982.
9. Stenlake, JF: Ions, cyclic nucleotids, cholinergy: In: Advances in Pharmacology and Therapeutics, ed by J.B. Stoclet. Oxford, Perganon Press, 1979.
10. Martin-Smith, M: Rational elements in the development of superior neuromuscular blocking agents. Chapter 12, In: Drug Design, ed by E.J. Ariens. New York, Academic Press, 1971.
11. Quevauviller, A, Huu-Laine, F: Sur la toxicite et le pouvoir curarisant du chlorure du malouetine. Am Pharmac Franc 18:678, 1960.
12. Savarese, JJ, Kitz, RJ: The quest for a short-acting nondepolarizing neuromuscular blocking agent. Acta Anaesth Scan (Suppl 53), 43-58, 1973.
13. Hewett, CL, Savage, DS: 2 , 16 , - Diaminoandrostanes. British Patent 1, 138, 605,(1965).

13a. Buckett, WR, Hewett, CL, Savage, DS: Pancuronium bromide and other steroidal neuromuscular blocking agents containing acetylcholine fragments. J Med Chem 16:1116-1124, 1973.

14. Savage, DS, Sleigh, T, Carlyle, I: The emergence of ORG NC45...from the pancuronium series. Br J Anaesth 52:35-39, 1980.
15. Durant, NN, Marshall, IG, Savage, DS et al: The neuromuscular and autonomic blocking activities of pancuronium, ORG NC45 and other pancuronium analogues in the cat. J Pharm Pharmacol 31:831-837, 1979.
16. Savarese, JJ, Ali, HH, Antonio, RP: The clinical pharmacology of metocurine: dimethyl-tubocurarine revisited. Anesthesiology 47:277-284, 1977.

Figure 1

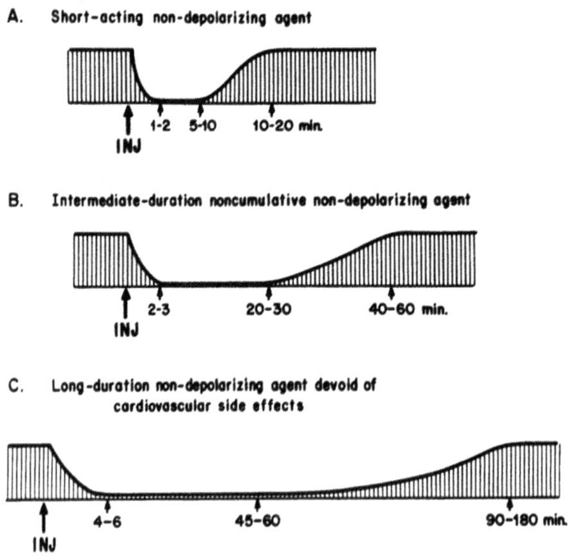

Fig 1 In an editorial written seven years ago, 3 hypothetical new relaxants which might be clinically useful were described. Drug A; a nondepolarizing relaxant with rapid onset and short duration of effect, would abolish the twitch, as diagramed at left, within less than 2 minutes and show complete recovery within 20 minutes or less. If this drug also produced little or no side-effect, it would constitute an "ideal" relaxant. Drug B at left has now been supplied by the introduction into clinical trials of atracurium (BW33A) and Vecuronium (ORG NC45). Although no drugs resembling "A" are at present in clinical trial, there is a good possibility for the development of such a drug in the near future. Drug C, an agent particularly useful for long operations and for intensive care use, should also be available, possibly as several different products, within a relatively short time.

Figure 2

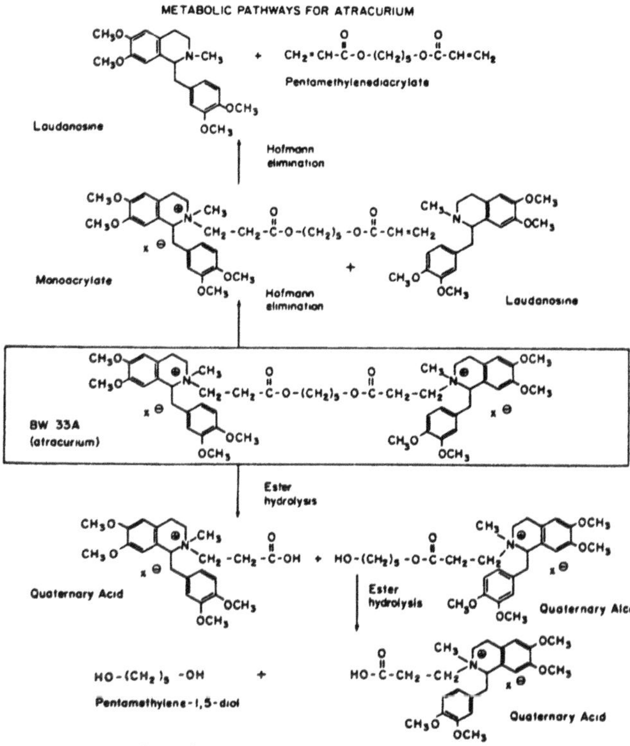

Fig 2 Proposed metabolic pathways for atracurium (BW33A), center of figure. The major pathway is Hofmann Elimination, a pH and temperature-dependent spontaneous rupture of the quaternary groups. The molecule was designed to undergo this chemical reaction which does not depend on organic biological processes. The drug is supplied as refrigerated solution at pH 3.5. When injected into the patient at 37°, a proton dissociates from the carbon α to the carbonyl carbon atom (β to the quaternary nitrogen), setting up electron shifts which result in disruption of the molecule into the metabolites which are shown. Atracurium also undergoes ester hydrolysis (probably enzymatic, but not catalyzed by plasma cholinesterase). The mechanism is favored at acidic pH. Since all of the metabolites of atracurium are pharmacologically inactive, it shows the least cumulative property in man of any known relaxant.[4,6]

Figure 3

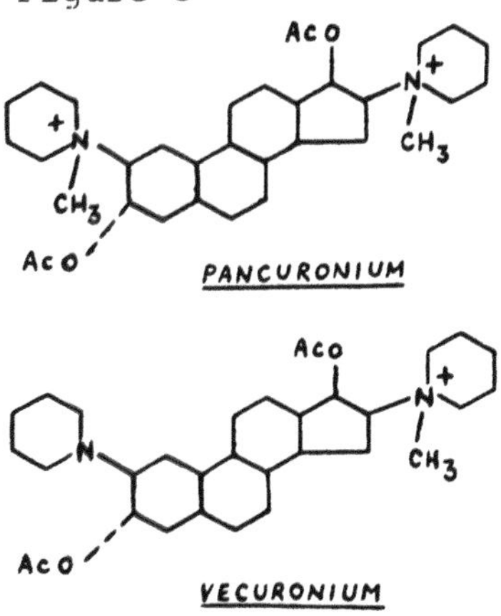

Fig 3 Comparative structures of pancuronium and Vecuronium (ORG NC45). The removal of the methyl quaternizing group at the 2-piperidino substitution reduces the vagolytic effects of pancuronium by a factor of 20.[15] Thus, the new drug vecuronium shows little or no cardiovascular effect. The same slight chemical change increases the lipophilic character of the molecule, making the bile its principal route of elimination.[8]

Figure 4

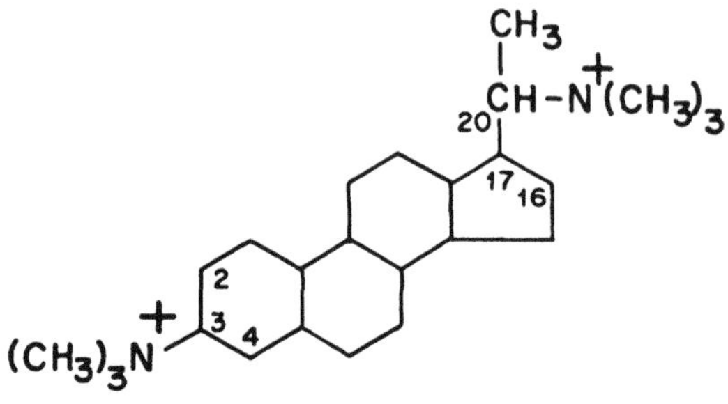

Malouétine

Fig 4 The chemical structure of malouetine, a naturally-occurring bi-quaternary steroidal molecule. This substance, the active principle of a poison prepared from a native plant source by inhabitants of the Belgian Congo (Zaire) was the first steroidal neuro muscular blocking drug ever discovered,[11] and led to the synthesis of many steroidal relaxants, ultimately to pancuronium and vecuronium.

Table 1
Comparative Pharmacokinetics of Pancuronium and Vecuronium in Normal Subjects and in Patients in Renal Failure[7]

Group	n	$T_{1/2}\alpha$ (min)	$T_{1/2}\beta$ (min)	V_{ss} (ml/kg^{-1})	Cl (mlmin^{-1})
Normal (pancuronium)	7	12.5±4.2	132.5±24.9	261.1±45.7	122.9±41.4
Renal failure (pancuronium)	10	12.1±8.6	257.3±128.2	295.9±158.3	53.0±15.7

Group	n	$T_{1/2}\alpha$ (min)	$T_{1/2}\beta$ (min)	V_{ss} (ml/kg^{-1})	Cl (mlmin^{-1})
Normal (ORG NC45)	4	8.5±4.0	79.5±13.6	194.3±41.3	227.5±37.5
Renal failure (ORG NC45)	5	10.5±4.8	97.1±37.7	238.7±62.6	176.1±34.2

Table 2
Comparative Urinary and Biliary Elimination of Pancuronium and ORG NC45 (Vecuronium) in Rats[8]

Rat	Urine (% of dose unchanged in urine after 12 hr)†	Bile (% of dose unchanged in bile after 7 hr)‡
ORG NC45		
1	3.9	
2	13.6	
3	5.0	
	(7.5±5.3)	
7		47.8
8		41.2
9		48.0
		(45.7±3.9)
Pancuronium		
4	90.1	
5	85.7	
6	78.5	
	(84.8±5.9)	
10		4.0
11		4.2
12		2.2
		(3.5 ±1.1)

NEW INTRAVENOUS ANESTHETIC DRUGS: ETOMIDATE AND MIDAZOLAM

J.G. REVES

New intravenous drugs hopefully are better than existing compounds. Intravenous anesthetics ideally provide hypnosis, amnesia, analgesia, without toxicity. There are two intravenous drugs whose release by the FDA is imminent. One is etomidate which is old, having been available for many years in Europe and the other is midazolam which is young and still being investigated worldwide. The following discussions review pertinent pharmacology of these drugs, some of which appear in Table 1 below.

Table 1.

COMPARISON OF ETOMIDATE AND MIDAZOLAM

	Etomidate	Midazolam
Dosage	.2-.3 mg/kg	.175-.30 mg/kg
Therapeutic Index (LD_{50}/ED_{50}-Animals)	26	200
Hypnosis	excellent	good
Amnesia	?	excellent
Analgesia	no	no
Pain on Injection	moderate	no
Thrombophlebitis	some	no
Onset	10-30 sec	30-90 sec
Acute Tolerance	no	?
Awakening	3-5 min	3-10 min
Elimination ½ life	29-75 min	78-132 min
Protein Binding	75%	96%
pKa	4.2	6.1
Respiratory Depression	mild (very transient)	mild (transient)
Cardiovascular Depression	no	slight

Data from references 1-11

ETOMIDATE

Etomidate was synthesized in 1965 by Godefroi and coworkers in the Janssen Pharmaceutica laboratory. The drug is a carboxylated imidazole, and it is most commonly compared with rapid acting barbiturates with which it shares many properties. Early laboratory studies demonstrated the very rapid hypnotic effect of etomidate, as well as a greater safety margin compared to thiopental and other rapid acting hypnotics (6). The speed of anesthetic induction with etomidate equals thiopental, but etomidate has a 5-fold greater therapeutic index (i.e. LD_{50}/ED_{50}) in animals, indicating that the drug should be safer for clinical practice. In our laboratory we found etomidate to have a safety margin four times greater than thiopental (12).

Etomidate is available and widely used in clinical practice in many countries throughout the world. From a combined series of 4,763 cases published in 1978, many of the clinical advantages and disadvantages of etomidate are reviewed (17). Etomidate is as rapid and short-acting as thiopental (8,13,14). Pharmacokinetic studies reveal that thiopental does have a longer elimination half-life (Table 2) (3,8,13,14). Etomidate is hydrolized in human liver, and apparently does not have an active metabolite. The drug is relatively less protein bound than other induction agents (75%). Because of rapid distribution, etomidate is well suited to continuous infusion methods for the maintenance of constant anesthetic depth (15). Because of the relative short elimination half-life and rapid plasma clearance there should be little etomidate accumulation if given by continuous infusion.

Induction with etomidate (.3 mg/kg) has been complicated by pain on injection and involuntary movements variously described as muscle twitches to seizures (7,16,17). Ghoneim has convincingly demonstrated that the movements are myoclonic and not associated with epileptiform EEG patterns (17). The incidence of venous pain reported with induction varies from 10%-50% in patients (7,16) but is less common with the new formulation containing 35% propylene glycol (18). However, the new formulation has a significant incidence of thrombophlebitis (up to 23% of patients) (9). Because of the pain with injection and the myoclonic movements during induction, anesthesiologists generally have rated thiopental or methohexital superior as an anesthetic induction agent.

Etomidate has little cardiopulmonary depression. Respiratory depression occurs with etomidate as reflected by slight arterial CO_2 retention in premedicated patients (10), and a significant incidence of apnea (7,16). Etomidate like thiopental produces a decrease in respiratory rate and minute volume, but the decrease in both are significantly greater with thiopental (11). Hemodynamic changes induced by etomidate are also minimal. Invasive hemodynamic studies in premedicated, healthy (19) and cardiac diseased patients (10) reveal a marked stability with etomidate induction. Although recent investigations have shown few hemodynamic changes with thiopental induction in healthy man (20,21), etomidate appears to produce even less changes, making it a potentially useful induction agent in patients with cardiovascular instability.

The presence of valvular heart disease may influence the hemodynamic responses to etomidate. Whereas most patients can maintain their blood pressure, patients who have both aortic and mitral valvular heart disease have significant decreases of 17 to 19% in systolic and diastolic blood pressure (22,23) and decreases of 11% and 17% in $\overline{PAP}$ and $\overline{PAO}$, respectively (23). Cardiac index in patients who have valvular heart disease and received 0.3 mg/kg either remained unchanged (22) or decreased 13%. There was no difference in response to etomidate between patients who had aortic valve disease and those who had mitral valve disease (23).

The cardiovascular effects of etomidate are not significantly altered by the simultaneous administration of other anesthetic drugs, though this has not been systematically studied with all drugs. The administration of 66% N_2O in oxygen has little effect on changes after induction with etomidate (24), nor does the presence of basal neurolept anesthesia (except possibly on contractility). Etomidate (0.3 mg/kg) reduced dP/dt 18% in patients anesthetized with neurolept drugs, but there was no change in either heart rate or blood pressure (25). Systemic blood pressure (14%), systemic vascular resistance (17%), and dP/dt (9%) decreased when etomidate 0.3 mg/kg was given to normal patients anesthetized with 0.3% halothane in 66% N_2O/O_2 (26). Wauquier and co-investigators anticipated the widespread clinical use of etomidate in their investigation comparing the effects of etomidate and thiopental in hypovolemic dogs (27). In a hemorrhagic shock model, dogs were bled to a mean arterial pressure of 40-45 mm Hg and then given either etomidate (1 mg/kg) or thiopental (10 mg/kg). There was significantly more hemodynamic depression in the thiopental group and increased survival in the etomidate group. Whether this is true in humans is not known, but certainly clinical evidence suggests that etomidate might be useful in hypovolemic patients.

There are certain indications for etomidate where its advantages outweigh the risks. Emergency uses include situations in which rapid induction is essential. Patients who have hypovolemia, cardiac tamponade, or low cardiac output probably represent the population for whom etomidate is better than other drugs, with the possible exception of ketamine. The fact that the hypnotic effect is brief means that additional analgesic and/or hypnotic drugs must be administered. Etomidate offers no real advantage over most other induction drugs for fit patients undergoing elective surgical procedures.

MIDAZOLAM

Midazolam is a water soluble, short lasting benzodiazepine synthesized in the United States laboratories of Hoffman-LaRoche in 1975. Formulated in an acid medium (pH 3.5), the compound is water soluble, but at pH above 4 it becomes lipid soluble. The rather unique pH dependent solubility accounts for the water solubility _in vitro_, and its lipid solubility (rapid anesthetic property) _in vivo_. Aqueous solubility obviates the necessity to dissolve the compound in organic solvents as must be done with diazepam.

Laboratory investigations proved that midazolam shared the prominent pharmacodynamic effects of other benzodiazepines. These include hypnotic, anticonvulsive, muscle relaxant and anxiolytic properties. In Table 2, the effects of midazolam and diazepam are compared. In general, midazolam is more potent and shorter-acting than diazepam. With specific regard to receptor CNS affinity, midazolam is approximately 2-fold greater than diazepam. Both equally affect gamma-aminobutyric acid (GABA), an inhibitory CNS transmitter, thought to be important in the mechanism of benzodiazepine action. With regard to cardiopulmonary effects in unanesthetized dogs, hypnotic dosages of 2, 4, and 10 mg/kg produced minor changes in hemodynamics, and arterial and venous blood gases (28), demonstrating a remarkable degree of safety.

Table 2.

COMPARISON OF PHARMACOLOGIC EFFECTS OF MIDAZOLAM AND DIAZEPAM

EFFECT	RESULT	DURATION
Anticonvulsant	M 2-4 X > D	M < D
CNS affinity	M 2 X > D	——
Muscle relaxation	D 2 X > D	M > D
GABA inhibition	M = D	——
Inhibition of discharge cerebellar neurons	M = D	D > M

Where M = Midazolam, D = Diazepam

Clinical studies show that midazolam may be used for sedation (29), premedication (30), and anesthesia induction (1,31) and, midazolam in unpremedicated, healthy patients is approximately 1½ times as potent as diazepam (1). Its onset of action is slightly more rapid than diazepam (1), but the duration of hypnotic effect after a single injection is short (6-19 min) (2,32). There is some evidence that males may be more susceptible to midazolam (32), but the reasons for this are not known. Pharmacokinetic studies in normal male volunteers reveal that the serum half-life (β t½) of midazolam is 1.3-2.2 hours (2), at least 10-fold shorter than diazepam (3). The drug is metabolized in the liver and at present there is no evidence of an active metabolite as is found with diazepam (desmethyldiazepam). Midazolam causes transient respiratory depression and apnea in some cases (33,34). In equipotent dosages midazolam and diazepam cause similar inhibition to a CO_2 challenge (4). On the basis of pharmacokinetic data, it is reasonable to predict that the respiratory depression will be shorter with midazolam than diazepam. Invasive hemodynamic studies in premedicated patients with ischemic heart disease anesthetized with midazolam show a transient decrease in blood pressure and systemic vascular resistance, with maintenance of cardiac index and slight increases in heart rate (5,35). These changes are very similar to diazepam (5) and unaffected by the addition of N_2O (36). Compared to thiopental (3 mg/kg), midazolam (.3 mg/kg) decreases blood pressure more because of greater decreases in systemic vascular resistance (37). Hemodynamic stability in healthy men has been reported over a 4-fold increase dosage schedule of .15, .3 and .6 mg/kg (38), similar to the large safety margin found in animals (28) (see Table 1).

Midazolam offers no advantage over thiopental for induction of anesthesia in healthy patients, but does appear to be superior for maintenance of anesthesia whether it be for short (33) or longer operations (39). Because of the short half-life of midazolam and the relatively rapid awakening (Table 1), it has been used in short operations in which the aim is to have patients "street-fit" which can be achieved by 4 hours following anesthesia and operation (33). Retrograde amnesia (40) and less nausea and vomiting are significant advantages of midazolam over thiopental. Midazolam compared with thiopental for maintenance of balanced anesthesia, requires less supplemental administration of narcotic and hypnotic drugs and fewer postoperative side effects (39). Because of cardiopulmonary stability, midazolam may be a good agent for poor risk patients, but this use has not been well documented. It appears that there may be more cardiovascular depression with midazolam than with diazepam. Midazolam will be a welcome benzodiazepine because of its short action and water solubility. It will be used for premedication, endoscopy sedation, cardioversion, anesthesia induction and anesthesia maintenance. It may also be used for sedation in a variety of intensive care settings.

Conclusion

Etomidate is a promising drug for use when rapid anesthesia induction and stable hemodynamics are required. Midazolam is much more versatile than etomidate. It, like diazepam, may be used as a sedative, hypnotic, induction agent, and anticonvulsant. The significant advantage of etomidate over thiopental is hemodynamic stability even in hypovolemic conditions and midazolam's advantage over diazepam are water solubility and rapid plasma clearance. Both drugs are welcome additions to the anesthesia formulary.

Acknowledgment

The author thanks the personnel at Janssen Pharmaceutica, particularly George Griffiths and Stan Rowe and at Hoffman-LaRoche Dr. Ilhan Tuzel and Jay Miller; all have provided useful information in preparing this report.

REFERENCES

1. Reves JG, Corssen G, Holcomb C. Comparison of two benzodiazepines for anesthesia induction: midazolam and diazepam. Can Anaesth Soc J 1978;25:211-214.
2. Brown CR, Sarnquist FH, Canup CA, et al. Clinical, electroencephalographic and pharmacokinetic studies of a water-soluble benzodiazepine, midazolam maleate. Anesthesiology 1979;50:467-470.
3. Ghoneim MM, Korttila K. Pharmacokinetics of intravenous anaesthetics: implications for clinical use. Clin Pharmacokinet 1977;2:344-372.
4. Forster A, Gardaz JP, Suter PM, et al. Respiratory depression by midazolam and diazepam. Anesthesiology 1980;53:494-497.
5. Samuelson PN, Reves JG, Kouchoukos NT, et al. Hemodynamic responses to anesthetic induction with midazolam or diazepam in patients with ischemic heart diesase. Anesth Analg 1981;60:802-809.
6. Janssen PAJ, Niemegeers CJE, Marsboon RPH. Etomidate, a potent non-barbiturate intravenous hypnotic. Intravenous etomidate in mice, rats, guinea pigs, rabbits and dogs. Arch Int'l Pharmacodyn Ther 1975;241:92-132.
7. Schuerman SV, Dom J, Dony J, et al. Multinational evaluation of etomidate for anesthesia induction: conclusions and consequences. Anaesthesist 1978;27:52-59.
8. Van Hamme MJ, Ghoneim MM, Ambre JJ. Pharmacokinetics of etomidate, a new intravenous anesthetic. Anesthesiology 1978;49:274-277.
9. Zacharias M, Clarke RFJ, Dundee JW, et al. Venous sequelae following etomidate. Br J Anaesth 1979;51:779-783.
10. Gooding JM, Weng JT, Smith, et al. Cardiovascular and pulmonary responses following etomidate induction of anesthesia in patients with demonstrated cardiac disease. Anesth Analg 1979;58:40-41.
11. Daehlin L, Gran L. Etomidate and thiopentone: a comparative study of their respiratory effects. Curr Therap Res 1980;27:706-713.
12. Kissin I, McGee T, Smith LR. The indices of potency for intravenous anesthetics. Can Anaesth Soc J 1981;28:585-589.
13. Ghoneim MM, Van Hamme MJ. Pharmacokinetics of thiopentone: effects of enflurane and nitrous oxide anesthesia in surgery. Br J Anaesth 1978;50:1237-1242.
14. Christensen JH, Andreasen F, Jansen JA. Pharmacokinetics of thiopentone in a group of young women and a group of young men. Br J Anaesth 1980;52:913-918.
15. Booij LHDJ, Rutten JMJ, Crul JF. Anesthesia with a constant infusion of etomidate in adult man. Acta Anaesth Belg 1978;29:165-170.
16. Fragen .RJ, Caldwell N, Brunner EA. Clinical use of etomidate for anesthesia inductoin: a preliminary report. Anesth Analg 1976;55:730-733.
17. Ghoneim MM, Yamada T. Etomidate: a clinical electroencephalographic comparison with thiopental. Anesth Analg 1977;56:479-485.
18. Fragen RJ, Caldwell N. Comparison of a new formulation of etomidate with thiopental - side effects in awakening times. Anesthesiology 1979;50:242-244.
19. Gooding JM, Corssen G. Effect of etomidate on the cardiovascular system. Anesth Analg 1977;56:717-719.
20. Becker KE, Tonnesen AS. Cardiovascular effects of plasma levels of thiopental necessary for anesthesia. Anesthesiology 1978;49:197-200.
21. Seltzer JL, Gerson JI, Allen FB. Comparison of the cardiovascular effects of bolus vs incremental administration of thiopentone. Br J Anaesth 1980;52:527-530.

22. Kettler D. Sonntag H, Wolfram-Donath U, et al. Haemodynamics, myocardial function, oxygen requirement, and oxygen supply of the human heart after administration of etomidate. In: Doenicke A. ed. Anaesthesiology and Resuscitatoin. New York: Springer Verlag, 1977:81-94.
23. Colvin MP, Savege TM, Newland PE, et al. Cardiorespiratory changes following induction of anaesthesia with etomidate in patients with cardiac disease. Br J Anaesth 1979;51:551-556.
24. Firestone S, Kleinman CS, Jaffe CC, et al. Human research and noninvasive measurement of ventricular performance: an echocardiographic evaluation of etomidate and thiopental. Anesthesiology 1979;51:S22.
25. Hempelmann G, Piepenbrock S, Hempelmann W, et al. Influence of althesine and etomidate on blood gases (continuous PO-monitoring) and hemodynamics in man. Acta Anaesth Belg 1974;25:402-412.
26. Patschke D, Bruckner JB, Eberlein HJ, et al. Effects of althesin, etomidate and fentanyl on haemodynamics and myocardial oxygen consumption in man. Can Anaesth Soc. J 1977;24:57-69.
27. Wauquier A, Hermans C, Van den Broeck W., et al. Resuscitative drug-effects in hypovolemic-hypotensive animals. Part 1: comparative cardiovascular effects of an infusion of saline, etomidate, thiopental or pentobarbital in hypovolemic dogs. Unpublished Observations.
28. Reves JG, Mardis M, Strong S. Cardiopulmonary effects of midazolam. Ala J Med Sci 1978;15:347-351.
29. Conner JT, Katz RL, Pagano RR, et al. RO 21-3981 for intravenous surgical premedication and induction of anesthesia. Anesth Analg 1978;57:1-5.
30. Vinik HR, Reves JG, Wright D. Premedication with intramuscular midazolam: a prospective randomized double blind controlled study. Anesth Analg (in press).
31. Fragen RJ, Gahl F, Caldwell NA. Water soluble benzodiazepine RO 21-3981 for induction of anesthesia. Anesthesiology 1978;49:41-43.
32. Forster A, Gardaz JP, Suter PM, et al. IV Midazolam as an induction agent for anaesthesia: a study in volunteers. Br J Anaesth 1980;52:907-911.
33. Fragen RJ, Caldwell NJ. Recovery from midazolam used for short operations. Anesthesiology 1980;53:S11.
34. Sarnquist FH, Mathers WD, Brock-Utne J, et al. A bioassy of a water-soluble benzodiazepine against sodium thiopental. Anesthesiology 1980;52:149-153.
35. Reves JG, Samuelson PN, Lewis S. Midazolam maleate induction in patients with ischemic heart disease: hemodynamic observation. Can Anaesth Soc J 1979;26:402-409.
36. Samuelson PN, Reves JG, Dole K, et al. Midazolam-N_2O induction in ischemic heart disease patients. Anesthesiology 1979;51:S104.
37. Al-Khudhairi D, Whitwam JG, Chakrabarti MK, et al. Haemodynamic effects of midazolam and thiopentone during induction of anaesthesia for coronary artery surgery. Br J Anaesth 1982;54:831-835.
38. Melvin MA, Johnson BH, Quasha AL, et al. Induction of anesthesia with midazolam decreases halothane MAC in man. Anesthesiology 1980;53:S10.
39. Reves JG, Vinik R, Hirschfield AM, et al. Midazolam compared with thiopentone as a hypnotic component in balanced anesthesia: a randomized, double-blind study. Can Anaesth Soc J 1979;26:42-49.
40. Reves JG. Benzodiazepines. In: Hug C, ed. Pharmacokinetics of Anesthetic Drugs. (in press)

THE NEW OPIOIDS

THEODORE H. STANLEY, M.D.

Until the last decade narcotics (opioids) were used by anesthesiologists as premedication drugs, as supplements during anesthesia with other agents and as post-operative analgesics.[1] In the last decade it has become recognized that narcotics may also provide significant advantages when used in larger doses, as anesthetics.[1-5] The most important initial report suggesting that narcotics could be anesthetics was that of Lowenstien and colleagues, which was published in December of 1969 in the New England Journal of Medicine.[2] In that article the authors indicated that one-half to 3 mg/kg of morphine would produce complete anesthesia and, in patients breathing oxygen who had no cardiovascular problems, little change in any of the cardiovascular variables which were measured, including cardiac output, systemic vascular resistence, arterial blood pressure, central venous pressure, pulse rate, and left ventricular work. In a group of patients with severe aortic valve disease, the same authors found that morphine anesthesia was associated with an increase in cardiac output and a decrease in systemic vascular resistance.

After an initial enthusiasm, many clinicians utilizing the "high" dose morphine technique became disenchanted with the drug as an anesthetic.[1,3] The most important reasons for this were the significant cardiovascular problems which occurred in many patients who were not gravely ill. These cardiovascular problems included hypotension, hypertension, bradycardia, tachycardia,marked increases in intra-operative and post-operative blood volume requirements, and myocardial depression when morphine was combined with other agents.[1,3,6,7] In addition to cardiovascular problems, clinicians had problems secondary to incomplete amnesia and profound postoperative respiratory depression. As a result, many began to modify the high dose morphine anesthetic technique by utilizing lower doses of morphine plus a variety of supplements. Use of the supplements changed the characteristics of morphine and, by and large, morphine plus supplementation with virtually any compound was found to be cardiovascular depressant.[1,7-9] Incomplete amnesia after morphine also raised the question of whether narcotics could ever be anesthetics.

In the last 5 years the synthetic opioid, fentanyl, has enjoyed an enormous amount of popularity.[10-14] The reason for this is related to studies in the late 1970's which suggested that anesthetic doses of fentanyl had most of the advantages of morphine but less of its disadvantages.[1,5,10] Advantages of high dose fentanyl anesthesia include: greater cardiovascular stability, particularly during induction of anesthesia but also during operation, little or no evidence of histamine release,[15] less evidence of venovasodilitation than morphine and, as a result, no increase in blood volume requirements intra-operatively and postoperatively, and significantly less postoperative respiratory depression.[1,5,10,16] In addition, some studies showed that large doses of fentanyl also did not result in elevations in antidiuretic hormone,[17] plasma cortisol,[11] or the circulating catecholamines.[11] These observations suggested that large doses of fentanyl were significantly different from any other anesthetic previously used for open heart or other major operative procedures.

The use of fentanyl as a complete anesthetic has become well established in open heart surgery and many other surgical procedures. In spite of its advantages, high doses of fentanyl, 75 to 150 ug/kg plus oxygen, does have some disadvantages.[1] Its onset of action is not as fast as a standard anesthetic induction agent such as thiopental.[1,16] Induction of anesthesia is often associated with an incidence of chest wall or total body muscle rigidity,[16,19] and, on occassion, there are hemodynamic evidences of incomplete suppression of the sympathetic nervous system, i.e. hypertension and tachycardia.[16,18] In addition, while respiratory depression is less than morphine, patients are not often able to resume normal spontaneous ventilation at the conclusion of operation.[5,10,16]

Recent experiments accomplished first in Holland and, more recently, in the United States, indicate that some of the newer cogeners of fentanyl, specifically sufentanil and alfentanil, may provide advantages over fentanyl as a complete anesthetic or even as an anesthetic supplement.[16,20-32] Of the new agents it appears that sufentanil is the most exciting as a complete anesthetic.[16,22,23] First of all, sufentanil has a therapeutic index for analgesia which is in the range of 25 to 30,000.[33] This compares quite favorably with the the therapeutic index of fentanyl, which is 270. In addition, in studies performed in Holland and subsequently repeated in the United States, it has been demonstrated that anesthetic induction can be accomplished somewhat faster with sufentanil, without incurring any additional side effects, e.g. an increase in the incidence of chest wall regidity or less evidence of cardiovascular stability.[16] Patients anesthetized with equipotent doses of fentanyl and sufentanil have been shown to have less hypertension intraoperatively with sufentanil than fentanyl and, as a consequence, to require less supplements during operation.[16] In addition, recovery seems to be somewhat faster with sufentanil than with fentanyl.[3] There are data which suggest that sufentanil is removed from the blood stream and probably also from the central nervous system faster than is fentanyl.[34]

An interesting spin-off of the comparison studies with sufentanil and fentanyl was the recognition that patients taking propranalol preoperatively required significantly less sufentanil for unconsciousness and the entire operation than patients not taking propranalol.[35] In addition, those patients taking propranalol and anesthetized with sufentanil had a much lower incidence of hypertension and therefore required intraoperative supplements less frequently than those not taking propranalol.

Initial studies suggested that both sufentanil and alfentanil used in anesthetic doses might be more effective in blocking increases in the stress responding hormones, particularly during cardiopulmonary bypass, than equivalent or even higher doses of fentanyl.[36] Subsequent studies have demonstrated that only some of the stress responding hormones are better blocked with sufentanil and alfentanil than fentanil.[22,37]

Alfentanil, which is a third as potent as fentanyl and has a third the duration of action of fentanyl, has been shown to also have a more rapid onset of action.[24-29] This suggests that alfentanil may have use as an anesthetic induction agent. Initial comparative studies evaluating alfentanil versus thiopental, etomidate and midazolam as induction agents suggest that alfentanil produces anesthesia almost as rapidly as thiopental and more rapidly than midazolam.[29,38] Alfentanil also produces little change in cardiovascular dynamics, not only during induction of anesthesia but also following endotracheal intubation.[29,38] Unfortunately almost all other available anesthetic induction agents are not analgesics, and as a result none of them can block the increases in blood pressure and heart rate that usually accompany endotracheal intubation immediately after induction. Profound cardiovascular stability after endotracheal intubation is considered by many to be a marked advantage of alfentanil over virtually all other anesthetic induction agents.[29,38] Although accompanied by a higher incidence of rigidity, there seem to be no other significant side effects of alfentanil as an anesthetic induction agent.

An additional advantage of alfentanil as an induction agent is a marked reduction in inhalation anesthetic requirements for up to 2 hours or more following anesthetic induction. It also appears that patients in the recovery room are more comfortable and require analgesics significantly less frequently following alfentanil induction when compared to induction with thiopental. Alfentanil may also have a place as a supplement during standard nitrous oxide-narcotic type of anesthesia. Its advantages as such would primarily be its rapid onset of activity and short duration of action. Unfortunately, this necessitates that the drug be given very frequently. Unpublished data (de Lange S, personal communication) suggest that alfentanil is best given as a continuous infusion when used in combination with nitrous oxide. At the end of the operative procedure the infusion is terminated and recovery is remarkably rapid.

Lofentanil and carfentanil are two new pure agonist narcotics that may have a place in anesthesia of the future. Advantages of these agents include their enormously high therapeutic indices, potential safety as sole narcotic anesthetics and supplements and extreme potency. These two agents, which are more potent and of longer duration than fentanyl, are undergoing initial animal experimentation in the United States and in Europe. The early findings (Stanley TH, unpublished data) suggest that anesthesia with these agents may be able to be accomplished via topical application (to mucous membranes), transcutaneous passage of the drugs, inhalation of nebulized mists or oral ingestion as well as via the more standard intravenous, intramuscular or subcutaneous routes.[39]

REFERENCES

1. Stanley TH: The pharmacology of intravenous narcotic anesthetics. In Anesthesia, Edited by Miller RD, New York, Churchill Livingstone, 1981
2. Lowenstein E, Hallowell P, Levine FH, et al: Cardiovascular response to large doses of intravenous morphine in man. N Engl J Med 281:1389-1393, 1969
3. Lowenstein E: Morphine "anesthesia" - A perspective. Anesthesiology 35:563-565, 1971
4. De Castro J: Analgesic anesthesia based on the use of fentanyl in high doses. Anesthesia vigile et suvigile 1:87-166, 1977
5. Stanley TH, Webster LR: Anesthetic requirements and cardiovascular effects of fentanyl-oxygen and fentanyl-diazepam-oxygen anesthesia in man. Anesth Analg 57: 411-416, 1978
6. Stanley TH, Gray NH, Stanford W, et al: The effects of high-dose morphine on fluid and blood requirements in open-heart procedures. Anesthesiology 38:536-541, 1973

7. McDermott RW, Stanley TH: The cardiovascular effects of low concentrations of nitrous oxide during morphine anesthesia. Anesthesiology 41:89-91, 1974
8. Stoelting RK, Gibbs PS: Hemodynamic effects of morphine and morphine nitrous oxide in valvular heart disease and coronary artery disease. Anesthesiology 38:42-52, 1973
9. Stanley TH, Bennett GM, Loeser EA, et al: Cardiovascular effects of diazepam and droperidol morphine anesthesia. Anesthesiology 44:255-258, 1975
10. Lunn JK, Stanley TH, Eisele JH, et al: High dose fentanyl anesthesia for coronary artery surgery: plasma fentanyl concentrations and influence of nitrous oxide on cardiovascular responses. Analg (Cleve) 58:390-395, 1979
11. Stanley TH, Berman L, Green O, et al: Plasma catecholamine and cortisol responses to fentanyl-oxygen anesthesia for coronary artery operations. Anesthesiology 53:250-253, 1980
12. Bovill JG, Sebel PS: Pharmacokinetics in high-dose fentanyl: A study in patients undergoing cardiac surgery. Brit J Anaesth 52:795-801, 1980
13. Robinson S, Gregory GA: Fentanyl-air-oxygen anesthesia for litigation of patent ductus artery ligation in preterm infants. Anesth Analg 60:331-334, 1981
14. Sebel PS, Bovil JG, Wauquier A, et al: Effects of high dose fentanyl anesthesia on the electroencephalogram. Anesthesiology 55:203-211, 1981
15. Rosow CE, Moss J, Philbin DM, et al: Histamine release during morphine and fentanyl anesthesia. Anesthesiology 56:93-96, 1982
16. de Lange S, Stanley TH, Boscoe M, et al: Comparison of sufentanil-O_2 and fentanyl-O_2 anesthesia in man. Anesthesiology 56:112-118, 1982
17. Stanley TH, Philbin DM, Coggins CH: Fentanyl-oxygen anaesthesia for coronary artery surgery: cardiovascular and antidiuretic hormone responses. Can Anaesth Soc J 26:168-172, 1979
18. Waller JL, Hug CC, Nagle DN, et al: Hemodynamic changes during fentanyl-oxygen anesthesia for aortocoronary bypass operations. Anesthesiology 55:212-217, 1981
19. Hill AB, Nahrwald MD, de Rosayro AM, et al: Prevention of rigidity during fentanyl-oxygen induction of anesthesia. Anesthesiology 55:452-454, 1981
20. Rolly G, Kay B, Cocks R: A double blind comparison of high doses of fentanyl and sufentanil in man. Influence on cardiovascular, respiratory and metabolic parameters. Acta Anaesth Belg 30:247-254, 1979
21. Sebel PS, Bovill JG: Cardiovascular effects of sufentanil anesthesia: A study in patients undergoing cardiac surgery. Anesth Analg (Cleve) 61:115-119, 1982
22. Sebel PS, Bovill JG, Fiolet J, et al: Hormonal responses to sufentanil anesthesia. Anesth Analg (Cleve) 61:214-215, 1982

23. Eriksen J, Berthelsen P, Ahn NC, et al: Early response to central hemodynamics to high doses of sufentanil or morphine in dogs. Acta Anaesth Scand 25:33-38, 1981
24. Niemegeers CJE, Janssen PAJ: Alfentanil, a particularly short-acting intravenous narcotic analgesic. Drug Development and Research 1:83-88, 1981
25. Brown JH, Pleuvry B, Kay B: Respiratory effects of a new opiate analgesic (R 39209) in the rabbit: Comparison with fentanyl. Brit J Anaesth 52:1101-1106, 1980
26. Kay B, Pleuvry B: Human volunteer studies of alfentanil (R 39209), a new short-acting narcotic analgesic. Anaesthesia 35:952-956, 1980
27. Kay B, Stephenson DK: Alfentanil (R 39209): Initial clinical experience with a new narcotic analgesic. Anaesthesia 35:1197-1201, 1980
28. Van Leeuwen L, Deen L: Alfentanil, a new potent and very short-acting morphinomimetic for minor operative procedures: A pilot study. Anaesthetist 30:115-117, 1981
29. Nauta J, Koopman D, Spierdijk J, et al: Alfentanil, a new narcotic anesthetic induction agent. Anesth Analg 61:267-271, 1982
30. Kay B: Postoperative pain relief. Use of an on-demand analgesia computer (ODAC) and a comparison of the rate of use of fentanyl and alfentanil. Anaesthesia 36:949-951, 1981
31. de Lange S, Stanley TH, Boscoe MJ: Alfentanil-oxygen anaesthesia for coronary artery surgery. Brit J Anaesth 53:1291-1296, 1981
32. de Lange S, de Briujin N, Stanley TH: Alfentanil-oxygen anesthesia: Comparison of continuous infusion and frequent bolus techniques for coronary artery surgery. Anesthesiology 55:A 43, 1981
33. De Castro J: Practical applications and limitations of anaesthesia. A review. Acta Anaesth Belg 3:107-128, 1976
34. Bovill JG, Sebel PS, Blackburn CL, et al: Kinetics of alfentanil and sufentanil: A comparison. Anesthesiology 55:A 174, 1981
35. Stanley TH, de Lange S, Boscoe MJ, et al: The influence of chronic pre-operative beta-adrenergic blocker therapy on intraoperative cardiovascular dynamics and narcotic requirements in patients with coronary artery disease. Can Anaesth Soc J 29:319-324, 1981
36. de Lange S, Boscoe MJ, Stanley TH, et al: Antidiuretic and growth hormone responses during coronary artery surgery with sufentanil-oxygen and alfentanil-oxygen anesthesia in man. Anesth Analg 61:434-438, 1982
37. de Lange S, Stanley TH, Boscoe M, et al: Catecholamine and cortisol responses to high dose sufentanil and alfentanil-O_2 anesthesia during coronary artery surgery. Anesth Analg 61:177-178, 1982
38. Nauta J, de Lange S, Koopman D, et al: Anesthetic induction with alfentanil: Comparison with thiopental, midazolam and etomidate. Can Anaesth Soc J (In Press)
39. Port JD, Stanley TH, Sterrey EM: Narcotic inhalation anesthesia. Anesthesiology 57:A 344, 1982

COMPARATIVE PHARMACOLOGY OF VOLATILE ANESTHETICS

ROBERT K. STOELTING, M.D.

Currently used volatile anesthetics (halothane, enflurane, and isoflurane) can have differing pharmacologic effects on 1) ventilation 2) circulation 3) central nervous system physiology and 4) the neuromuscular junction. Likewise, the physical and chemical characteristics of these drugs vary resulting in predictable differences in the rate of induction and recovery from anesthesia as well as the extent of biotransformation (Table 1). Meaningful information regarding the comparative pharmacology of inhaled anesthetics mandates their comparison at equal potent concentrations (equivalent MAC values) in patients who are similar with respect to age and general health. These types of data are available from healthy volunteers and serve as the foundation for establishing comparative differences between volatile anesthetics (1). However, it must always be appreciated that the surgical patient with co-existing disease, concomitant drug therapy and altered intravascular fluid volume can respond differently from the healthy volunteer despite exposure to identical concentrations of a volatile anesthetic.

Table 1.	HALOTHANE	ENFLURANE	ISOFLURANE
MAC	0.75	1.68	1.15
BLOOD/GAS	2.4	1.9	1.4
MOLECULAR WEIGHT	197.4	184.5	184.5
VAPOR PRESSURE (20C)	244	172	240
PRESERVATIVE	Yes	No	No
STABILITY IN SODA LIME	No	Yes	Yes
REACTS WITH METAL	Yes	No	No
BIOTRANSFORMATION (percent of absorbed dose)	20	2.4	0.17

VENTILATION

Volatile anesthetics produce dose-dependent depression of ventilation characterized by elevations of the $PaCO_2$ (Figure 1) (1) and depression of the ventilatory response to carbon dioxide (2). In healthy volunteers 1 to 1.2 MAC enflurane produces a greater increase in the $PaCO_2$ than do equivalent concentrations of halothane or isoflurane. Substitution of nitrous oxide for an equivalent portion of the volatile anesthetic results in less increase in the $PaCO_2$ than that produced by the volatile anesthe tic alone. The beneficial effect of nitrous oxide on limiting the increase in $PaCO_2$ is seen with all three volatile anesthetics but the greatest impact is present when nitrous oxide is used to replace an equivalent amount of enflurane (2).

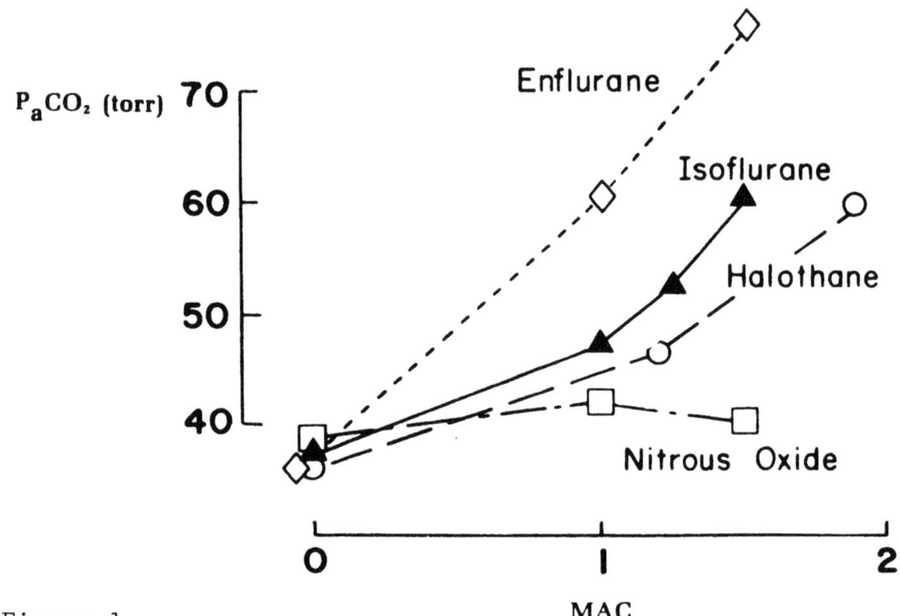

Figure 1.

Recovery from the ventilatory depressant effects of volatile anesthetics can be demonstrated after 5 hours of administration. Evidence for this recovery is a smaller rise in the $PaCO_2$ and less rightward shift of the carbon dioxide response curve after 5 hours of administration compared with that produced by the same anesthetic concentration at 1 hour of administration. Recovery is seen with all three volatile anesthetics, but the greatest change is present with enflurane (Table 2) (2).

Table 2. ARTERIAL PCO_2

ENFLURANE	1 HOUR	5 HOURS
1 MAC	61 torr	46 torr
2 MAC	Apnea	61 torr

The bronchodilating effects of halothane are a frequent determinant in the selection of this drug for administration to patients with increased airway resistance. However, animal evidence demonstrates that isoflurane is equally effective in attenuating increases in airway resistance (3).

CIRCULATION

Volatile anesthetics administered to volunteers during controlled ventilation of the lungs to maintain normocarbia produce dose-dependent reductions in blood pressure (Figure 2) (1). Enflurane decreases the mean arterial pressure more than halothane or isoflurane. Substitution of nitrous oxide for an equivalent amount of the volatile anesthetic results in evidence of sympathomimetic stimulation characterized by increased blood pressure, cardiac output, systemic and pulmonary vascular resistance. These sympathomimetic changes are most evident when nitrous oxide is added to halothane, intermediate with isoflurane and not detectable with enflurane.

Volatile anesthetics differ with respect to changes produced in heart rate (1). Compared with awake values, the heart rate is unchanged during administration of 1 to 2 MAC halothane. Over the same dose range, isoflurane increases heart rate about 20 percent above awake levels. Enflurane is the only volatile anesthetic that produces dose-dependent elevations in heart rate (40 percent increase at 1.5 MAC).

Volatile anesthetics produce dose-dependent reductions in cardiac output (1). Isoflurane, 1 MAC, does not change cardiac output from awake levels compared with a 20 to 30 percent reduction associated with the administration of halothane and enflurane. Calculation of stroke volume demonstrates that the decreased cardiac output produced by enflurane and halothane is due to decreased myocardial contractility. Isoflurane reduces stroke volume but the mild increase in heart rate is sufficient compensation to maintain the cardiac output. Isoflurane may differ from other volatile anesthetics by virtue of an inherent ability to preferentially depress activity of the parasympathetic nervous system. The net effect is a predominance of sympathetic nervous system activity.

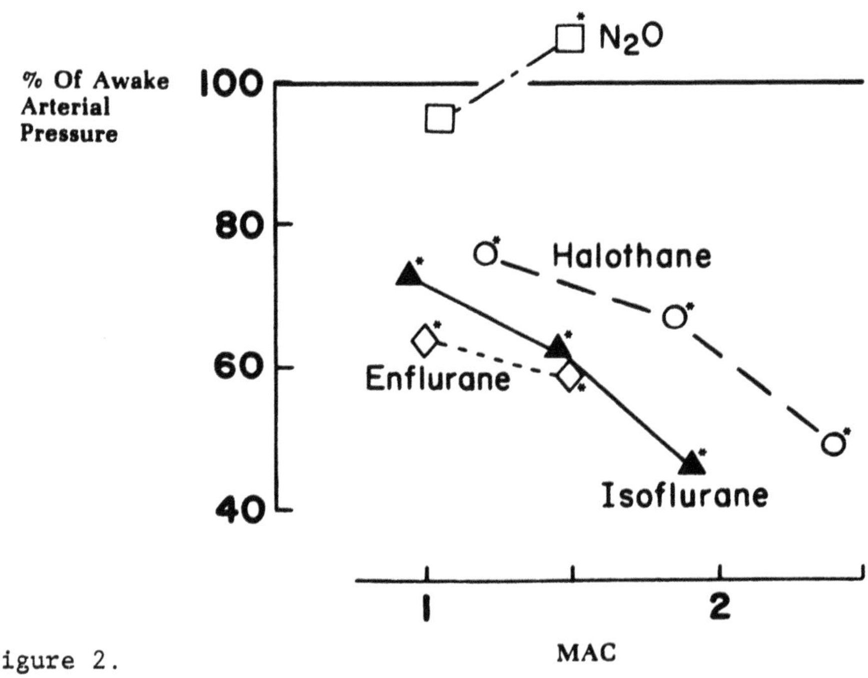

Figure 2.

Isoflurane and to a lesser extent enflurane reduce the systemic vascular resistance while no change in this calculated value is produced by the administration of halothane (1). A two to three-fold increase in skeletal muscle blood flow is a unique characteristic of isoflurane and contributes to the reduction in systemic vascular resistance produced by this drug. The magnitude of reduction in systemic vascular resistance produced by isoflurane is less when nitrous oxide is substituted for an equivalent amount of isoflurane.

Recovery from the circulatory effects produced by volatile anesthetics is evident after 5 hours of administration. For example, compared with measurements after 1 hour of administration the same measurements at 5 hours reveal similar reductions in blood pressure but the cardiac output is less depressed, the heart rate is further increased and the systemic vascular resistance is further reduced. Recovery is most evident during the administration of halothane and enflurane and is insignificant for isoflurane.

Stability of cardiac rhythm is influenced by the specific volatile anesthetic that is being administered. For example, the submucosal dose of epinephrine necessary to produce ventricular irritability is 2.1 ug/kg during the administration of halothane and 6.7 ug/kg in the presence of isoflurane (4). This difference in dysrhythmic threshold may reflect the ability of isoflurane (enflurane too) to accelerate conduction of the cardiac impulse through the atrioventricular node and bundle of His. Conversely, halothane slows conduction of the cardiac impulse favoring the appearance of an ectopic focus or the development of a re-entry phenomena.

The impact of prior beta-adrenergic block on the circulatory responses produced by volatile anesthetics has important implications. Animal evidence indicates that beta-adrenergic block acutely produced by intravenous propranolol has no effect on the magnitude of changes in blood pressure or cardiac output produced by isoflurane (5). In a similar study, the blood pressure reduction produced by 1 MAC halothane in the presence of beta-adrenergic block was similar to the decrease produced by 1.5 MAC halothane in the absence of beta-adrenergic block. Compared with isoflurane and halothane, circulatory changes produced by enflurane are exaggerated the most by beta-adrenergic block.

CENTRAL NERVOUS SYSTEM

Volatile anesthetics increase cerebral blood flow in a

dose-dependent manner (1). For example, cerebral blood flow and autoregulation are not significantly altered by the administratio of 0.6 MAC halothane, enflurane or isoflurane. At 1.1 MAC, cerebral blood flow is increased nearly three-fold by halothane while the magnitude of increase is much less in the presence of enflurane and halothane. In patients with space-occupying intracranial lesions, a drug-induced increase in cerebral blood flow can result in abrupt elevations of the intracranial pressure Institution of hyperventilation for 10 minutes ($PaCO_2$ 25 to 30 torr) before introduction of halothane or enflurane into the inspired gases attenuates the increase in intracranial pressure that occurs if these drugs are administered in the presence of normocarbia or simultaneously with the institution of hyper-ventilation (6). In contrast to halothane and enflurane, the administration of isoflurane simultaneously with the onset of hyperventilation attenuates drug-induced increases in intracranial pressure (7).

Volatile anesthetics have differing effects on the electro-encephalogram. For example, enflurane produces spike and wave activity particularly when greater than 2 MAC is administered. In contrast, the chemical isomer of enflurane, isoflurane, does not produce seizure activity. Furthermore, isoflurane has anticonvulsant properties in animals. Isoflurane is also unique in that it is capable of producing electroencephalographic silence at a clinically acceptable concentration (2 MAC) (1).

NEUROMUSCULAR JUNCTION

Volatile anesthetics enhance the effects of nondepolarizing muscle relaxants but the magnitude of effect is drug-specific (Table 3) (1). Isoflurane is the only anesthetic that alters the response produced by succinylcholine. Isoflurane and enflurane (1.25 MAC) exert direct effects on the neuromuscular junction as evidenced by failure to sustain an evoked response to tetanic stimulation (160 Hz) despite the absence of neuro-muscular blockers. The direct effects of isoflurane and enflurane on the neuromuscular junction suggests these drugs could be used as inhaled muscle relaxants in combination with traditional nondepolarizing neuromuscular blockers. It may be possible to produce adequate relaxation for surgery with reduced doses of a nondepolarizing muscle relaxant that would have insignificant neuromuscular junction effects after excretion of the volatile anesthetic. Indeed, reductions in twitch height during a continuous infusion of d-tubocurarine are directly related to the end-tidal concentration of enflurane (8).

Table 3. DOSE OF MUSCLE RELAXANT (mg/m^2) TO DEPRESS TWITCH 50 PERCENT

	HALOTHANE*	ENFLURANE*	ISOFLURANE*
SUCCINYLCHOLINE	5.1	4.9	3.4
d-TUBOCURARINE	5.6	1.6	1.7
PANCURONIUM	0.49	0.29	0.27

*1.25 MAC

REFERENCES

1. Eger EI. Isoflurane (Forane). A compendium and reference. Ohio Medical Products 1981.
2. Lam AM, Clement JL, Chung DC, Knill RL. Respiratory effects of nitrous oxide during enflurane anesthesia in humans. Anesthesiology 1982;56:298-303.
3. Hirshman CA, Edelstein G, Peetz S, Wayne R, Downes H. Mechanism of action of inhalational anesthesia on airways. Anesthesiology 1982;56:107-11.
4. Johnston RR, Eger EI, Wilson C. A comparative interaction of epinephrine with enflurane, isoflurane and halothane in man. Anesth Analg 1976;55:709-12.
5. Philbin DM, Lowenstein E. Hemodynamic consequences of the combination of isoflurane anesthesia (1 MAC) and beta-adrenergic blockade in the dog. Anesthesiology 1975;42:567-73.
6. Adams RW, Gronert GA, Sundt TM, Michenfelder JD. Halothane, hypocapnia, and cerebrospinal fluid pressure in neurosurgery. Anesthesiology 1972;37:510-7.
7. Adams RW, Cucchiara RF, Gronert GA, Messick JM, Michenfelder JD. Isoflurane and cerebrospinal fluid pressure in neurosurgical patients. Anesthesiology 1981;54:97-9.
8. Gencarelli PJ, Miller RD, Eger EI, Newfield P. Decreasing enflurane concentrations and d-tubocurarine neuromuscular blockade. Anesthesiology 1982;56:192-4.

PREVENTION AND TREATMENT OF INTRAOPERATIVE MYOCARDIAL ISCHEMIA

J. H. TINKER, M.D.

RISK AND RISK MANAGEMENT

The diagnosis of significant or critical coronary artery disease (CAD) is not easily made during the preoperative visit. If a patient has had a prior myocardial infarction (MI), you have no good idea whether there are any other critical stenoses present. It is possible that the previous MI obliterated the area that was at risk and now, although the patient may have considerably less cardiac reserve than previously, there is little danger of developing a new MI. It is much more likely that patients who have suffered prior MI's have multiple coronary vessel involvement. All that can be done is to delineate known risks in such patients and balance said risks against the necessity of the procedure vs the risk of not doing it. Steen et al,[1] in 1978, reporting on 74,000 patients operated on at the Mayo Clinic between the years 1974 and 1975, found that approximately 6 percent of the 587 patients who had suffered documented prior MI's, suffered another MI during the first 7 days after anesthesia and surgery. Further, almost 70 percent of those MI's resulted in death. Recent myocardial infarction poses an even greater problem. Steen et al[1] reported that if the MI had occurred within three months of the anesthesia and surgery, the risk of a new MI was approximately 30 percent, dropping to about 15 percent if the MI was between 3 and 6 months old. Recently, Rao and El-Etr[2] reported on 97 patients who underwent emergency or semi-emergency operations within 6 months of an MI, many of them within 3 months. They reported that, with invasive monitoring placed before induction and left in place several days postoperatively, with aggressive use of beta blockers, vasodilators, antidysrhythmics and other aggressive measures, they were able to reduce the incidence of reinfarction of only 7.8 percent in the patients with recent infarctions less than 3 months old and to only 3.4 percent in the patients with infarctions 3-6 months old. This represents a major improvement over the results previously published by many authors including Steen et al.[1] Further, most if not all of the patients of Rao and El-Etr[2] were emergent or semi-emergent cases. This is the first report that begins to document our long-cherished idea that aggressive hemodynamic monitoring and resultant adjustments during surgery (and following surgery) really do make a difference in outcome. This is a most encouraging and exciting prospect, if it can be confirmed.

What other patients besides those who have suffered a prior MI are at risk? The only known cause of angina pectoris is myocardial regional supply/demand imbalance. On the other hand, clearly not all that is chest pain has anything to do with the heart whatsoever. Careful histories should be taken in patients who have undiagnosed chest pains, especially after age 40. Suspicion that CAD may be present should be thought of as follows. If the patient's chest pain is in fact due to his/her heart, then CAD or coronary spasm is present to a sufficient degree to cause at least the beginnings of myocardial ischemia. This means that it is serious enough to demand a competent cardiologic workup. To dismiss chest pain as being likely due to "heart burn", "gallbladder" and one or another muscle ache syndromes, is playing a deadly game. Often, anesthetists are fooled into playing this game by patients themselves who also are denying the cardiac possibilities. This author knows of two massive intraoperative MI's, one fatal, which were directly due to the anesthetist's, during preoperative rounds, believing the patient's explanation for epigastric pain.

Other patients who are likely to have hidden CAD include female diabetics. The extent to which their small vessels are involved is often unknown. Further, their activity levels may be low enough so that chest pain doesn't often occur. Chest pain referral patterns may be disrupted by diabetic neuropathies. In short, the female diabetic, especially if she has peripheral vascular disease of any sort, should wave a red flag about the possibility of CAD.

What about heavy smokers? A 55-year-old man with a 40 pack-year history of smoking is so likely to have CAD that it can almost be considered concomitant. In a recent series we have investigated over 1500 patients who underwent coronary artery bypass. Nearly 80% are or were smokers.

Can we manage this risk? Despite the Rao and El-Etr[2] report, we would still not wish to perform elective surgery within 6 months of an MI. To put some numbers on this, the patient with a less than 3-month-old MI, scheduled for TUR of the prostate is a common occurrence. In our's and the literature's experience, this patient has approximately a one in three chance of having a new MI in 7 days following anesthesia and surgery and if that MI occurs, the death rate will be 50-70%. All told, that means that this individual has a 15% chance of dying from his heart plus whatever risks the TUR adds. If the TUR is semi-emergent because of recurrent obstructions, we would think it logical, although there is no evidence either way, to ask the surgeon to do only a minimal obstruction-relieving procedure. Knowledge of these numbers can therefore aid in risk management.

Prevention

Preventing intraoperative myocardial ischemia means somehow blunting that individual's response to a truly massive stimulation (namely surgery) and its resultant catecholamine release both into blood and at adrenergic nerve endings. It means blunting that response at its peak while not that many minutes later it also means not producing such myocardial depression as to produce severe hypotension-induced subendocardial ischemia. Let us break this down into several topics.

Work - Hydraulic work is mean pressure times flow. Thus, for the cardiovascular system, cardiac work is, roughly, mean arterial pressure times cardia output. Although this is the "business end" i.e. the energy output, it accounts for only 5 to 15% of the total energy consumed by the myocardium. Even the inefficient gasoline engines of a few years ago in Detroit automobile were over 20% efficient. Today's more efficient gasoline engines are in the neighborhood of 30% efficient with the deisel engines sometimes topping 40% thermal efficiency. The important message here is that our long-cherished ideas that if we can provide hemodynamic stability we will prevent myocardial ischemia may need modification. If we provide such hemodynamic stability and the "hemodynamics" that we monitor with our most sophisticated tools today are really only the determinants of external work (plus heart rate), then we are only monitoring 15% or less of the total MVO_2. We hope that the rest follows the external work component but in fact there is evidence that it does not necessarily do so.[3] Worse, it is logical, but unproven, that the lowest possible total myocardial oxygen demand might be best in terms of prevention of myocardial ischemia. At first glance this seems like a great idea, but on careful thought it may not be true. The lowest possible overall myocardial oxygen demand may result in such low coronary artery perfusion pressures that the "rich" begin to steal from the "poor" and, gradually, myocardial ischemia develops beyond stenotic vessels. Work is pressure times flow. Increasing pressure at constant flow causes dramatic and linear increases in myocardial oxygen demand. On the other hand, assuming constant heart rates for these examples, increasing flow, even tripling it, at constant pressure, results in almost no increase in myocardial oxygen demand.[4] In other words, the heart is a much more efficient flow pump that it is a pressure pump. Deliberately placing additional afterload such as use of vasoconstrictors or aortic crossclamps, will cause a dramatic increase in myocardial oxygen demand. One of the most potent of these afterload increasers is surgical incision under too-light anesthesia.

Monitors as Preventatives - Thus, under "prevention" we come to monitors. The definition of a monitor, in my opinion, is that it should be a gadget that not only tells us when something is wrong, but gives us a way to fix it. We know ahead of time that we are going to subject our CAD patient, almost surely, to some, possibly great, increases in afterload. We need to monitor this patient's cardiac function to see how the myocardium handles said increases in afterload. If an aortic crossclamp is applied and wedge pressure increases substantially, we may or may not be dealing with myocardial ischemia. Certainly we are dealing with evidence of decreased myocardial compliance. Nonetheless, the monitor gives us knowledge that a perturbation has occurred and allows us to monitor its correction during vasodilator therapy. If such increases in end-diastolic pressure, monitored by wedge pressure, are promptly treated and corrected, then it may matter little which came first. It is possible that subendocardial ischemia resulted in ventricular dysfunction which in turn resulted in an elevation in the wedge pressure. It is also possible that the myocardium is merely adjusting to a new preload position in order to be able to respond to the added afterload and that in fact no subendocardial ischemia exists yet. Nonetheless, at this new preload position, the subendocardium may be subjected to a greater "squeeze". This is because the coronary arterial pressure drop across the myocardium is the mean arterial pressure in the epicardial arteries minus the subendocardial pressure. Raising the latter will of course decrease the pressure head available for perfusion of the subendocardium. Thus, when said "squeeze" occurs, even if the original elevation in preload was not due to actual ischemia, but rather to poor ventricular compliance, subendocardial ischemia may only be a few more beats away. Thus the monitor becomes a preventative.

Rate - The pioneering work of Loeb et al[5] has clearly shown us that human hearts subjected to the same increases in overall MVO_2 fared much worse when subjected to increases in MVO_2 via a rate (tachycardia) mechanism than they did at the same increases in MVO_2 brought about by an increase in afterload with the drug methoxamine. I said above that increasing afterload resulted in dramatic and virtually linear increases in MVO_2. Often, unless there is a decrease in ventricular compliance, as mentioned above, increases in MVO_2 (demand) will be accompanied by increases in supply because the pressure head has increased. The opposite is true for increases in heart rate. Now diastol time is decreased and it is during diastole that virtually 100% of subendocardial blood flow occurs. It is now widely accepted that preventing tachycardia is one of if not the single most important thing to do in order to try to prevent intraoperative myocardial ischemia. The patient who arrives in the operating room with a heart rate of 60 (often due to beta blocker therapy) may, because of surgical stimulation and rapid decline in beta blocke blood levels, be soon found to have a heart rate of 85. This is a large percentage increase. Does it represent a tachycardia? My answer to that is that it can never be known in any given patient just what the ischemia-inducin tachycardia threshold is. Some anesthetists have glibly advocated exercising these patients on treadmills preoperatively until they developed angina and then trying not to let the heart rate go above that level (minus a safety margin) during anesthesia. I hope this audience can see that we need to get much more sophisticated than this. Clearly, anesthetics change myocardial size and contractility and therefore may change pressure/flow/rate relationships. For example, it is possible indeed that some anesthetics may favor the "rich" and further hinder the "poor" postcritical stenotic areas of myocardial muscle. It is certainly logical that heart rates above 100 should not be tolerated in most patients with CAD. An exception to this would be the patient who is labeled as "CAD" but who in fact has end-stage ventricular failure at a high heart rate. This patient will not be able to increase stroke volume if you deliberately lower the rate. In fact, lowering the rate in this patient may be very difficult but if you accomplish it, you may accomplish the patient's demise because this patient has rate-dependent cardia output. It is not entirely fair to call these patients "CAD" patients because they are very different from the usual patient who has a reasonably sound myocardial muscle with poor blood supply.

Diagnosis and Treatment

When ST-segment depression occurs in an operating room setting, you have no choice but to make the diagnosis of intraoperative myocardial ischemia, realizing that it may be late. It is possible, though extremely unlikely in an operating room setting that coronary artery spasm will occur, accompanied by ST-segment elevation instead of depression. The reason this is so unlikely may be the same reason why the cerebral vasospasm which plagues neurosurgical patients postoperatively, rarely occurs in the operating room unless it is caused by local surgical stimulation. The vasodilating properties of anesthetics may play a role. "Garden variety" myocardial ischemia in the operating room is heralded by ST-segment depression, especially in the V5 lead. If circulatory hyperdynamism, characterized by tachycardia and/or hypertension, was recognized a few minutes earlier, treatment measures are already underway. These treatment measures should consist of, first and foremost, reducing heart rate. We would administer beta blocker, unless contraindicated (asthma, allergy) as our drug of first choice. We would use heart rate as our end-point and try to get the heart rate at least back down into the 70's. We would give 0.5 mg propranolol per bolus, would given our boluses 1-2 minutes apart and would not be afraid to administer total propranolol dosages in the region of 4-6 mg if needed. Usually, arterial pressure will also decrease. We would follow the beta blockade with a vasodilator, usually nitroglycerin. We try to titrate the nitroglycerin using wedge or PA diastolic pressure, reducing that value back toward control to try to minimize subendocardial "squeeze". Arterial pressure may become unacceptably low. Balancing beta blocker and vasodilator therapy is not easy. Beta blocker-vasodilator therapy thus seems a logical part of "balanced" anesthesia, even if CAD is not obviously present preoperatively.

Do not expect ST-segments to become isoelectric within two or three minutes after heart rate and pressure reduction. They may be depressed for many minutes, even an hour or so and still slowly improve. It is entirely possible that despite your best efforts, this patient's myocardium will go on to develop infarction. That infarction may be heralded by severe intractable hypotension and low cardiac output syndromes. A diagnosis of cardiogenic shock is unavoidable here. The treatment of cardiogenic shock should be aimed at improving myocardial supply and decreasing demand. This cannot be done with any inotrope/vasodilator combination known. There is no such thing, contrary to some written opinions, as a "pharmacologic balloon pump". If severe myocardial ischemia persists in the operating room with low cardiac output syndrome, the intra-aortic balloon pump should be resorted to if possible. You will need to "tide" your patient over with an inotrope/vasodilator combination. After we have tried dopamine/dobutamine, etc., we usually use epinephrine and nitroglycerin. Isoproterenol is clearly contraindicated because it dilates muscle beds, produces tachycardia and dysrhythmias, and may even lower mean arterial pressure.

What about the calcium entry blockers?[6,7] ST-segment depression does not have to be the first sign of myocardial ischemia. Frequent premature ventricular contractions, especially multifocal, and/or A-V block can be first signs of ischemia. If there is tachycardia, there is often a 'temptation to use verapamil. Verapamil has a very selective depressant effect on the A-V node. Ischemia-related first degree A-V block can be converted into complete block by even a small dose of verapamil. A complete block, in turn, may result in severe hypotension secondary to low output secondary to severe bradycardia. Thus, the verapamil may induce a vicious cycle which will make the myocardial ischemia worse. We believe that verapamil is probably better suited for the treatment of certain supraventricular tachydysrhythmias such as are seen during emergence from cardiopulmonary bypass. Nifedipine would seem to be more useful in treatment of intraoperative myocardial ischemia, because it does not have a selective effect on the A-V node, depresses MVO_2 and contractility, and causes peripheral vasodilation. It is associated with more reflex-induced tachycardia, however. Addition of beta blocker to nifedipine may obviate said tachycardia. This discussion is academic, however, because nifedipine is not available intravenously. Thus, our first line of defense during intraoperative myocardial ischemia is still beta blocker-vasodilator therapy. The persistent supraventricular tachycardias mentioned above can be seen with digitalis toxicity, rapid atrial fibrillation, low cardiac output syndromes following cardiopulmonary bypass. Verapamil can be very useful in these situations. We doubt that, as we gain experience with it we will find it more useful than propranolol during acute intraoperative myocardial ischemia. PR interval should be carefully monitored during its use and, if it appears to be lengthening, we would strongly advise against further dosage because complete AV block may be next.

Summary

With our most sophisticated monitors, we still can only monitor pressures flows, and calculate resistances, coupled with heart rate. We are not, by these means, monitoring the majority of overall MVO_2. Intra and postoperative MI's have occurred in patients in whom such external work indices were successfully held within narrow and acceptable limits. Still, with today's degree of sophistication, we do believe that avoidance of circulatory hyper- and hypodynamism, avoidance of tachycardia, prompt therapy for tachycardia with beta blockers, prompt therapy of hypertension with vasodilators, often nitroglycerin, and therefore sound minute-to-minute hemodynamic management both intra- and postoperatively will lead to reduction in incidence and severity of intraoperative myocardial ischemia and its consequences.

References

1. Steen PA, Tinker JH, Tarhan S: Myocardial reinfarction after anesthesia and surgery. JAMA 239:2566-2570, 1978
2. Rao TLK, Et-Etr A: Reinfarction following anesthesia in patients with myocardial infarction. In press, Anesthesiology
3. Tinker JH, Nugent M, Barash PG, Kay H: Cardiac O_2 use efficiency vs four anesthetics: halothane/enflurane better than fentanyl without beta blockade in swine. Anesthesiology 57:A18, 1982
4. Nugent M, Walls JH, Tinker JH, Harrison CE: Low O_2 cost if preload increase triples cardaic work. Anesthesiology 53:S111, 1980
5. Loeb HS, Saudye A, Croke RP, et al: Effects of pharmacologically-induced hypertension on myocardial ischemia and coronary hemodynamics in patients with fixed coronary obstruction. Circulation 57:41-46, 1978
6. McGoon MD, Vlietstra RE, Holmes DR, et al: The clinical use of verapamil. Proc Mayo Clin 57:495, 1982
7. Cohn JN, Editor, Calcium entry blockers in coronary artery disease. Am Heart Assoc Monograph No. 84. Circulation 65:I1-I59, 1981

TOXICITY OF LOCAL ANESTHETICS IN THE ADULT, FETUS AND NEWBORN

M. FINSTER, M.D.

With the growing popularity of regional anesthesia for the relief of pain in labor and delivery, there has been increasing interest in and concern about the effects of local anesthetics on the mother, fetus and the newborn. This interest has led to numerous studies relating to the pharmacokinetics of these drugs and to their potential toxic effects.

The passage of drugs across the placenta and their distribution into and ultimate removal from fetal tissues are influenced by a variety of factors. Of prime significance are the physicochemical properties of the compound in question. Equally important, however, are the pertinent anatomical features of the maternal circulation, the placenta, and the fetus, as well as hemodynamic and pharmacokinetic events within them.

PHYSICOCHEMICAL PROPERTIES

Foreign organic substances penetrate most cells as though the boundary had the characteristics of a lipoid membrane. Such a membrane is almost impenetrable by charged or ionized particles but is relatively permeable to unionized molecules, whose rate of transfer depends upon the lipid solubility of the molecule. All local anesthetics are highly soluble in lipids, particularly bupivacaine and etidocaine, two new long-acting drugs. Nitrogenous local anesthetics are weak bases and can occur in aqueous solutions partly as undissociated free bases and partly as dissociated cations. The ratio of these two moieties is of pharmacological importance, since it is the base that is believed to penetrate the tissue diffusion barriers, whereas the cation is considered to block conduction when in direct contact with the nervous tissue. Commonly used local anesthetics have pKa values ranging from 7.7 to 9.1. These values are sufficiently close to the blood pH, so that maternal or fetal acid-base imbalance should result in significant changes in the ratio of ionized to unionized fractions of the drug. Thus, in the acidotic fetus, the proportion of ionized drug is greater than in the healthy one.

Molecular size is also of importance. Assuming adequate lipid solubility, most unionized drugs of molecular weight less than 600 cross cell boundaries readily. Molecular weights of the commonly used local anesthetic drugs range from 220 for prilocaine to 325 for bupivacaine.

Local anesthetics in the maternal circulation traverse the placenta by simple diffusion, a process governed mainly by physicochemical factors in accordance with Fick's law. The rate of diffusion is a function of the concentration gradient of the substance between maternal and fetal blood, the surface available for transfer, and the thickness of the membrane.

FACTORS AFFECTING MATERNAL BLOOD LEVELS OF LOCAL ANESTHETICS

These factors include total dose, site of injection, addition of epinephrine to the solution, and rate of metabolism and excretion. For example, absorption of local anesthetics from the paracervical area appears to be more rapid than that from the epidural space owing to the greater vascularity of the area. All amide-linked local anesthetics have been detected in the maternal blood within minutes of their administration. Mepivacaine reaches peak concentrations in maternal blood within 25 - 40 minutes following a single epidural injection. The subsequent decline is sufficiently slow to account for maternal (and fetal) drug accumulation after repeated injections. This maternal accumulation can be reduced by the use of long-acting local anesthetics, such as bupivacaine or etidocaine, which require less frequent reinjection, or by use of drugs that are rapidly metabolized. Insignificant maternal blood levels have been demonstrated following the use of 2-chloroprocaine, an ester-type drug, which is hydrolyzed by plasma pseudocholinesterase ($T_{1/2}$ = 21 sec). Metabolism of this drug was seen even in plasma samples obtained from subjects with homozygous atypical cholinesterase, although at a slower rate ($T_{1/2}$ = 106 sec). Addition of epinephrine to local anesthetic solution will produce local vasoconstriction and may delay the uptake from the site of injection. However, because of potentially harmful effects of epinephrine in reducing uterine activity and blood flow, its use is controversial in obstetric anesthesia.

ANATOMICAL AND HEMODYNAMC FACTORS

Uterine blood flow increases steadily throughout pregnancy, reaching an average value of 500 to 700 ml per minute. Reduction in uteroplacental blood flow, from whatever cause, will result in decreased delivery of the drug to the fetus. A variable proportion of the umbilical vein blood perfuses the fetal liver and enters the inferior vena cava through the hepatic vein, and the remainder is shunted through the ductus venosus directly into the inferior vena cava. Consequently, a portion of any drug is strained through the liver before gaining access to the rest of the fetus. Furthermore, the drug undergoes progressive dilution during its transit to the arterial side of the fetal circulation, as blood in the umbilical vein becomes admixed with fetal venous blood from the gastrointestinal tract, from the lower extremities, from the head and upper extremities, and finally from the lungs. This unique pattern of the fetal circulation results in a delay in equilibration between fetal tissues and fetal blood mainfested by the persistent gradient in drug concentrations between the umbilical vein and the umbilical artery.

Distribution of fetal cardiac output may be altered by fetal hypoxemia and acidosis. Under these conditions, blood flow to the placenta and to the fetal brain, heart and adrenals increases substantially, while perfusion of the fetal lungs, kidneys, spleen, gut and carcass diminishes. Drug distribution in fetal tissues should follow similar patterns. Local anesthetics transmitted to the fetus may themselves affect its hemodynamic state. In pregnant ewes, infusion of lidocaine to the mother resulted in reduction of fetal cardiac output and umbilical blood flow, particularly in fetuses that were acidotic prior to the infusion.

FACTORS AFFECTING FETAL TISSUE UPTAKE

Any drug transferred across the placenta is carried to fetal tissues, where its uptake depends on the tissue-blood partition coefficient of the drug and the tissue perfusion. Uptake of lidocaine in fetal tissues was studied in pregnant guinea pigs following intravenous injection into the mother. Relatively high concentrations were found in fetal liver, myocardium and brain, demonstrating the rapid distribution to highly perfused fetal organs. The liver was the only organ in which lidocaine levels in the fetus exceeded those in the mother.

The importance of lipid solubility in the fetal tissue uptake of local anesthetics has recently been demonstrated in another study comparing the placental transfer of several local anesthetics in pregnant guinea pigs. The ratio of etidocaine or bupivacaine concentration between the fetal and the maternal blood was substantially lower than that found for lidocaine. However, the proportion of the injected dose recovered from fetuses over the first 60 mintues was remarkably similar for all three drugs studied. In contrast, the uptake of etidocaine or bupivacaine in the fetal myocardium, brain and liver was substantially greater than that of lidocaine. These relatively high tissue levels of long-acting agents in the fetus relate to the fact that bupivacaine is approximately ten times, and etidocaine fifty times, more soluble in lipids than is lidocaine. High protein binding of bupivacaine and etidocaine failed to limit their placental transfer.

METABOLISM AND EXCRETION IN THE FETUS AND THE NEWBORN

Experimental data gathered over the last few years indicate that the fetus and the newborn may be capable of metabolizing and excreting local anesthetics. For example, in plasma samples obtained from the human umbilical vessels at birth, 2-chloroprocaine was rapidly hydrolyzed, the half-life being approximately 43 seconds. Our detailed pharmacokinetic study of lidocaine in fetal and newborn lambs and adult sheep indicates that the metabolic clearance in the newborn is quite similar to, and the renal clearance is greater than, that in the adult. Nonetheless, the elimination half-life is more prolonged in the newborn. This prolongation is due to a greater volume of distribution and tissue uptake of the drug, the result being that at any given time the neonate's kidneys are exposed to a smaller fraction of the lidocaine accumulated in the body.

IS THE NEWBORN MORE SENSITIVE TO LOCAL ANESTHETICS THAN THE ADULT?

The answer to this question is dependent upon which symptom of toxicity one chooses as a criterion. Neonatal depression was noted in infants with umbilical vein levels of lidocaine or mepivacaine in excess of 2.5 to 3.0 µg per milliliter, which is approximately 50 percent of the toxic threshold of the adult. However, infants who were inadvertently intoxicated with mepivacaine during attempted caudal anesthesia stopped convulsing when their drug concentration fell below 8 µg per milliliter of blood, which is similar to the adult convulsive threshold. Finally, when lidocaine was infused intravenously into newborn and adult sheep, the doses required to produce convulsions, respiratory arrest, hypotension or circulatory collapse were greater in the newborn. Measurements of lidocaine concentrations in blood demonstrated that these toxic symptoms occurred at levels which were not significantly different between the newborn and the adult.

REFERENCES

1. Brown WU, Bell GC, Alper MH: Acidosis, local anesthetics and the newborn. Obstet Gynecol 48:27-30, 1976
2. Biehl D, Shnider SM, Levinson G, et al: Placental transfer of lidocaine: Effects of fetal acidosis. Anesthesiology 48:409-412,1978
3. O'Brien JE, Abbey V, Hinsvark O, et al: Metabolism and measurement of chloroprocaine, an ester-type local anesthetic. J Pharm Sci 68:75-78, 1979
4. Kuhnert BR, Kuhnert PM, Prochaska AL, et al: Plasma levels of 2-chloroprocaine in obstetric patients and their neonates after epidural anesthesia. Anesthesiology 53:21-25, 1980

5. Shnider SM, Way EL: The kinetics of transfer of lidocaine (Xylocaine[R]) across the human placenta. Anesthesiology 29:944-950, 1968
6. Finster M, Morishima HO, Boyes RN, et al: The placental transfer of lidocaine and its uptake by fetal tissues. Anesthesiology 36:159-163, 1972
7. Morishima HO, Finster M, Pedersen H, et al: Placental transfer and tissue distribution of etidocaine and lidocaine in guinea pigs. Abstracts of Scientific Papers, American Society of Anesthesiologists, 1975, pp 83-84
8. Brown WU, Bell GC, Lurie AO, et al: Newborn blood levels of lidocaine and mepivacaine in the first day of age following maternal epidural anesthesia. Anesthesiology 42:698-707, 1975
9. Ralston DH, Shnider SM: The fetal and neonatal effects of regional anesthesia in obstetrics. Anesthesiology 48:34-64, 1978
10. Morishima HO, Covino BG: Toxicity and distribution of lidocaine in nonasphyxiated and asphyxiated baboon fetus. Anesthesiology 54:182-186, 1981
11. Morishima HO, Finster M, Pedersen H, et al: Pharmacokinetics of lidocaine in fetal and neonatal lambs and adult sheep. Anesthesiology 50:431-436, 1979
12. Morishima HO, Pedersen H, Finster M, et al: Toxocity of lidocaine in adult, newborn and fetal sheep. Anesthesiology 55:57-61, 1981

ANESTHESIA FOR CESAREAN SECTION: REGIONAL AND GENERAL

CHARLES P. GIBBS, M.D.

Introduction

Anesthesia for cesarean section can be accomplished with either regional anesthesia or general anesthesia. When performed properly, both should provide safe, effective anesthesia for mother and infant.[1,2] Datta and Alper have recently written a comprehensive review of the topic.[3]

Before discussing anesthesia however, it is necessary to explain reasons for the current high cesarean section rate. Average rates are in the 13-16% range with some centers reporting rates less than 10% and others greater than 25%. These rates are markedly different from the 5-10% rates that prevailed in the 1960's. A recent Consensus Development Task Force on Cesarean Section found the following indications responsible, to the degrees indicated, for the increase in cesarean sections.[4]

1. Repeat cesarean section - 23.9%.
2. Dystocia - 23.9%.
3. Breech Presentation - 11.5%.
4. Fetal Distress - 10.3%.

The above figures indicate that electronic fetal monitoring leading to a more frequent diagnosis of fetal distress, is not the major contributor to increased rates. Rather, repeat cesarean section and dystocia are the primary causes. As long as the dictum, "Once a cesarean section, always a cesarean section" is espoused, the number of cesarean sections being performed on a repeat basis will increase as the number of primary cesarean sections increase. To slow this increase, many obstetricians are allowing selected patients who have had previous cesarean sections to undergo a trial of labor and vaginal delivery. To encourage this practice, The American College of Obstetricians and Gynecologists has published "Guidelines for Perinatal Care".[5] This document offers suggestions regarding anesthesia practice and personnel as well as the entire obstetric side of the problem. They suggest that anesthesia and obstetric personnel be present in-house whenever such a trial takes place. Because of the rather strict guidelines governing vaginal delivery following cesarean section, the larger reductions in rates will be seen primarily in the larger centers.

The other major indication for cesarean section is dystocia. The term "dystocia" is a relatively inexact term relating to the inability of the fetus to negotiate the birth canal. Reasons may be insufficient uterine contractions, inadequate bony pelvis, or an excessively large infant relative to the pelvis. These three features are occasionally referred to as the three "Ps": power, passage and passenger. Because some obstetricians believe this indication is used too frequently, The American College of Obstetricians and Gynecologists is also preparing a document addressing this indication. Thus, we may be seeing fewer cesarean sections performed on a repeat basis or for dystocia.

Although there is also some move to allow more breech presenting infants to deliver vaginally, the success of this movement is doubtful because gross morbidity and mortality figures support cesarean birth so very strongly.

GENERAL ANESTHESIA

Advantages. The advantages can be listed as follows:

1. Awake and unaware.
2. Total pain relief.

3. Little risk of drug depression when administered properly.

4. Optimum operating conditions.

Disadvantages

1. Asleep and unaware.
2. Husband less likely to be allowed in O.R.
3. Drug depression of fetus.
4. Cardiovascular changes of intubation.
5. Aspiration.
6. Difficult intubation.

The last two disadvantages represent significant hazards for the mother and are causing many obstetrical anesthesiologists to prefer and suggest regional anesthesia. Recent studies from England and Wales indicate that general anesthesia was responsible for thirty-nine maternal deaths during a three-year period, while regional anesthesia was responsible for only two.[6] Moreover, general anesthesia was the primary cause of mortality associated with cesarean section. Aspiration and failure to be able to intubate the trachea, along with inexperienced personnel, represented the vast majority of the problems associated with general anesthesia in these cases.[6] Although the United States does not have access to such data, anecdotal reports, as well as data from state maternal mortality committees, indicate that similar findings would prevail if such data were available for review.

Indications

Clinical situations in which general anesthesia may be more appropriate than regional anesthesia include the following:

1. Hypovolemia or hemorrhage.
2. Severe, acute fetal distress.
3. Patient refusal of or inability to cooperate for regional anesthesia.
4. Certain forms of heart disease that cannot tolerate hypotension, e.g. aortic stenosis.

5. Anesthesia personnel are inexperienced in providing regional anesthesia.

6. Any instance when regional anesthesia is contraindicated.

Technique

Although there are many individual variations on how to provide general anesthesia for cesarean section, usually the process is accomplished in a manner similar to the one outlined below:

1. Premedication: Atropine 0.4-0.6 mg or glycopyrrolate 0.2-0.3 mg I.M. or I.V.[7]

2. Antacids: Prophylactic use of antacids to reduce acidity of stomach contents is widely and appropriately accepted.[8] Because particulate antacids may produce rather extensive histologic and physiologic derangement,[9] clear nonparticulate antacids such as 0.3 M sodium citrate or Bicitra produce very little lung damage and are equally as effective as particulate antacids.[10,11,12] Unfortunately, 0.3 M sodium citrate is not commercially available in this country and must be prepared by the hospital pharmacies according to a specific formula[10]. However, Bicitra, a commercially available urinary alkalinizing agent, contains a comparable amount of sodium citrate and has recently been found innocuous when aspirated.[11]

3. Left uterine displacement (LUD): The uterus impinges on the inferior vena cava during the latter months of pregnancy preventing cardiac return and thus reducing cardiac output. The reduction in cardiac output may then lead to a reduction in uterine blood flow with or without obvious maternal hypotension. This phenomenon helps answer the frequently asked question, "What is the optimum time for delivery of the infant under general anesthesia?" Although several estimates have been suggested in the past, Crawford has provided an appropriate answer.[13] He studied two groups of patients, one in which LUD was practiced and one in which it was not. In the LUD group there was very little

difference in Apgar scores of infants related to anesthesia time. In the other group the incidence of low Apgar scores increased as the length of induction to delivery increased. Regarding the same topic, recent data indicate that it is not the induction of anesthesia to delivery interval that matters, but rather the uterine incision-delivery interval.[14] As this interval increases low Apgar scores increase.[14] It is during this interval that difficulties with the operation and excessive manipulation of uterine vessels occur as the length of the interval increases.

4. Preoxygenation: Always a good idea. Only 4-5 large breaths may be necessary.[15]

5. Precurarization: Some do not believe that this is necessary, and perhaps it isn't.[16] The reason for precurarization is to inhibit succinylcholine-induced muscle fasciculations which in turn raise intragastric pressure.[16a] However, during fasciculation, pressures above the lower esophageal sphincter may rise as much as intragastric pressures, thus minimizing risk from the increased intragastric pressure.[15] Also, pregnant patients appear to fasciculate very little following succinylcholine. Thus, the use of curare may serve only to make the succinylcholine less effective and the intubation more difficult.

6. Thiopental, 3-4 ml/kg, or ketamine, 1 ml/kg: Both of these agents have been used extensively as induction agents and have been shown to have very little, if any, effect on the newborn.[17,18] Ketamine has the advantage of possessing its own analgesia as well as providing somewhat better neurobehavioral scores.[19]
Also, Schultetus has recently shown that ketamine produces no greater and perhaps even less cardiovascular hyperactivity than does thiopental.[20]

7. Cricoid Pressure:[21] A simple maneuver to prevent regurgitation of stomach contents. It should always be applied immediately following the induction dose of thiopental or ketamine and not released until the

endotracheal tube is known to be in place and the cuff inflated.

8. Succinylcholine, 1-2 ml/kg: This drug does not cross the placenta in any significant clinical amount.

9. Intubation: The anesthetist must be skilled at performing rapid (crash) intubation. Aspiration does not occur only during mask anesthesia; it also occurs during difficult or delayed intubation attempts. Informal surveys of teaching hospitals and private hospitals indicate that the incidence of difficult or delayed intubations is approximately 5%. Cricoid pressure should not be released during a difficult or delayed intubation unless active retching occurs.[5]

10. Check for bilateral breath sounds: The tube must be in place before the operation begins.

11. Nitrous oxide/oxygen in a 50-50 mixture. Safe for mother and fetus.[22]

12. Halothane, 0.5% or enflurance, 0.5-1.0%: These two agents increase analgesia as well as decrease the amount of awareness. In these concentrations they do not promote uterine bleeding.[23,24]

13. Succinlycholine drip: Used to supplement this technique if coughing and bucking occur before delivery of the infant.

14. Once the infant is delivered, halothane or enflurane can be continued or a narcotic, such as fentanyl, will provide additional analgesia.

15. Oxytocin: 10-40 units per liter given as an intravenous infusion. When given as a bolus, this agent can produce marked vasodilitation and hypotension.[25]

16. Extubation: The patient is extubated awake. That is, she is responsive to oral command as well as being completely recovered from whatever muscle relaxation was used. Aspiration not only occurs at the time of induction of anesthesia but also during emergence.

17. Recovery Room: The patient is taken to any appropriately staffed and equipped recovery room. This

recovery room may be located in the obstetrical area of the hospital or may be in the general operating area. The most important requirement is that trained personnel be available to care for her during recovery from anesthesia.

Conclusion

General anesthesia, when administered properly, can provide effective and safe anesthesia for both mother and neonate. However, because aspiration and failure to be able to intubate represent significantly greater hazards to the mother than do the risks associated with regional anesthesia, an effort should be made to utilize the latter whenever feasible.

REGIONAL ANESTHESIA

Advantages. Regional anesthesia for cesarean section offers the following advantages:

1. Awake and participating.
2. Little risk of drug depression.
3. Little risk of aspiration.
4. Little risk of intubation difficulty.
5. Good neurobehavioral scores (see below)
6. Increased FIO_2.
7. Father in delivery room.

Disadvantages:

1. Awake and aware.
2. Inadequate block (choose surgeons and patients wisely).
3. Hypotension.
4. Total spinal.
5. Local anesthetic toxicity.
6. Contraindications.

Neurobehavioral scores represent a relatively new way of evaluating newborn infants.[26] Presumably, these scores reflect the functioning of a newborn's higher cortical centers as opposed to Apgar scores and acid-base values which evaluate only brain-stem function. In the last several years, this type evaluation has produced many reports in both the scientific and lay press. Briefly, the results can be summarized as follows:

1. Infants of mothers who receive regional anesthesia score better than those receiving general anesthesia.[19,27]

2. Ketamine, as an induction agent produces better scores than does thiopental.[19]

3. Narcotics produce lower scores.[28]

4. Bupivacaine and chloroprocaine produce better scores than lidocaine and mepivacaine.[26] Although these difference have been noted, it is important to recognize that a special committee gathered by the F.D.A. has declared that there are no long term effects on neurobehavioral performance or intelligence. Yet, strangely, the F.D.A. continues to require such tests on all new drugs for use in obstetrics. Finally, and perhaps most important,[14] Abboud et al have demonstrated convincingly that there really is no difference between lidocaine and mepivicaine and bupivacaine and chloroprocaine.[29] Hypotension, perhaps the most frequent complication of regional anesthesia, can occur in 25-75% of either spinal or epidural anesthesia - even when all prophylactic measures are taken.[1,2,30,31] The etiology is sympathetic blockade that causes vasodilitation and subsequently decreased cardiac return which leads to hypotension, decreased uterine blood flow and decreased maternal cerebral blood flow. To prevent hypotension, LUD is used after the patient has been given 1500-2000 cc of Ringer's lactate solution.[31,32] Ringer's lactate solution is chosen over D_5R/L because rapid intravenous administration of D_5R/L may produce hypoglycemia in the newborn.[33] (Infants insulin response to the glucose load outlives the glucose and hypoglycemia results at approximately two hours following birth). Another prophylactic measure is the administration of 25-50 mg of ephedrine IM.[30] A newer prophylactic measure using 5% albumin solution as a preloading fluid seems particularly effective but expensive.[34]

The treatment of hypotension includes placing the patient in Trendelenburg position in conjunction with LUD. More fluids are administered and, if necessary, ephedrine, 10-15 mg intravenously, is given.[33,34] Recently, Datta has indicated that immediate treatment with ephedrine of an initial 10 mmHg decline in blood pressure will preclude any significant hypotension.[35] When hypotension is treated promptly and effectively, little, if any harm comes to the healthy fetus.[35,36] However, if hypotension occurs in a patient with a compromised fetus, that fetus may be harmed.[37] Therefore, in these compromised patients, an albumin solution plus immediate treatment of even a small initial decline in blood pressure is indicated. Albumin is effective because it will stay in the intravascular space much longer than will crystalloid.[38]

Which local anesthetic? In the sixties and early seventies lidocaine and mepivacaine were the agents of choice. In the mid seventies chloroprocaine and bupivacaine were introduced and gained immense popularity. Chloroprocaine, an ester, was quickly metabolized, and had a short onset and duration. Bupivacine, an amide, was highly protein bound and thus less crossed the placenta. Both agents provided good sensory pain relief with little motor impairment. Also, perhaps most important - or at least most dramatic - these two local anesthetics allowed for better neurobehavioral scores in the newborns.[26] Recently however, they have been the subject of serious controversy. Chloroprocaine has been implicated as causing prolonged neurologic damage,[39,40,41] and reports substantiating or denying the charge have been numerous.[42,43,44,45,46] Although all regional anesthetic techniques may be capable of producing some neurologic damage in rare instances, the final answer as to whether or not 2-chloroprocaine is more prone to do so is not yet answered in this author's mind. If one chooses to use chloroprocaine for epidural anesthesia, guidelines as outlined by Covino et al[47] and Moore[48] should be followed.

Bupivacaine has also been tainted by being accused of producing cardiovascular depression at levels usually only toxic to the central nervous system.[49] There have been case reports, experimental studies and many anecdotal reports that tend to support or deny the contention that bupivacaine may be unusually cardiodepressant.[50,51,52] In the usual clinical report, an intravascular injection provokes a CNS reaction (convulsions) that is accompanied by cardiac depression to the degree that the patient cannot be resuscitated.[53] Thus, if this drug is used, three recommendations seem appropriate. 1) For the test dose, Moore[48] recommends that 3 ml of local anesthetic with 0.15 mg (1:200,000) of epenephrine be used. The epenephrine, if intravascular, will cause a rise in heart rate of approximately 30 beats per minute and thus alert one to the intravascular placement. 2) If a convulsion occurs, oxygenate, ventilate and remember that most will subside spontaneously and quickly. If not, the muscular aspects of the seizure can be terminated by succinylcholine. Drugs which are depressant to the heart should be avoided. 3) If cardiac compression becomes necessary, displacement of the uterus is mandatory to assure adequate cardiac return. Because of these rather serious concerns about these two agents, some authorities have opted to avoid either one or both of them. Many have chosen to return to lidocaine, which, after all the furor about neurobehavior scores has settled, has been convincingly exonerated.[29] Of course, another choice for regional anesthesia is the time tested spinal anesthesia.

Techniques

The following techniques for performing spinal anesthesia and lumbar epidural anesthesia are offered. Obviously, there are other techniques that are equally acceptable.

Spinal Anesthesia

1. Pre-operative antacids.
2. Explain procedure.

3. Lateral position.
4. Pre-hydrate with 1500-2000 cc R/L.
5. Vital signs. Monitor BP, EKG, heart sound.
6. Prepare and drape back.
7. Prophylactic ephedrine?.
8. Atraumatic tap.
9. Tetracaine: 7,8, or 9 mgm depending on height of patient.
10. Try for T_4-T_6 level:
    Position
    Frequent level checks.
11. Supine position
12. Frequent BP checks
13. If hypotension occurs: fluids, position, vasopressor.
14. Be there.

Lumbar Epidural- Much the same as for spinal except for the following:

1. Test dose: 3 ml 1.5% lidocaine, 3% chloroprocaine, or 0.75% bupivacaine with 1:200,000 epinephrine.[48]
2. 16-20 cc of 3% 2-chloroprocaine, 0.5%-7.5% bupivacaine or 1.5-2.0% lidocaine, all incrementally.
3. Precautions against and the treatment of hypotension the same as for spinal.

The above represents a general discussion of anesthesia for cesarean section. There has been no attempt made in this presentation to discuss anesthesia for cesarean section in patients with complicating diseases. For those patients, adaptations of the above techniques are needed to accommodate them to the particular disease.

REFERENCES

1. James FM, et al: A comparison of general anesthesia and lumbar epidural analgesia for elective cesarean section. Anesth Analg 56:228, 1977.
2. Magno R, Kjellmer I, Karlsson K: Anesthesia for cesarean section. III: Effects of epidural analgesia on the respiratory adaptation of the newborn in elective cesarean section. Acta Anaesth Scand 20:73, 1976.
3. Datta S, Alper MH: Anesthesia for cesarean section. Anesthesiology 53:142-160, 1980.
4. Cesarean Childbirth. Report of a Consensus Development Conference Sponsored by the National Institute of Child Health and Human Development, October 1981.
5. Guidelines for Vaginal Delivery After a Cesarean Childbirth. American College of Obstetricians and Gynecologist's Committee on Obstetrics: Maternal and Fetal Medicine, January, 1982.
6. Tomkinson J, Turnbull A, Robson G, et al: Report on confidential enquiries into maternal deaths in England and Wales 1973-75.
7. Baraka A, Saab M, Salem MR, et al: Control of gastric acidity by glycopyrrolate premedication in the parturient. Anesth Analg 56:642-645, 1977.
8. Roberts RB, Shirley MA: Reducing the risk of acid aspiration during cesarean section. Anesth Analg 53:373, 1974.
9. Gibbs CP, Schwartz DJ, Wynne JW, et al: Antacid pulmonary aspiration in the dog. Anesthesiology 51:380, 1979.
10. Gibbs CP, Spohr L, Schmidt D: The effectiveness of sodium citrate as an antacid. Anesthesiology 57:44, 1982.
11. Eyler SW, Cullen BF, Murphy ME, et al: Antacid aspiration in rabbits: A comparison of mylanta and bicitra. Anesth Analg 61:288, 1982.
12. Lahiri SK, Thomas TA, Hodgson RMH: Single-dose antacid therapy for prevention of Mendelson's Syndrome. Br J Anaesth 45:1143, 1973.
13. Crawford JA, Burton M, Davies P: Time and lateral tilt at cesarean section. Br J Anaesth 44:477, 1972.
14. Datta S, Alper MH, Brown WU, et al: Anesthesia for cesarean section: Importance of induction-delivery and uterine incision-delivery interval on neontal outcome. Abstracts of Scientific Papers, Annual Meeting. Park Ridge, Illinois, American Society of Anesthesiologists, 1978, pp 103-104.
15. Gold MI, Muravchick S: Arterial oxygenation during laryngoscopy and intubation. Anesth Analg 60:316-318, 1969.
16. Smith G, Dalling R, Williams TIR: Gastro-esophageal pressure gradient changes produced by induction of anaesthesia and suxamethonium. Br J Anaesth 50:1137, 1978.

16a. Miller RD, Way WL: Inhibition of succinylcholine-induced increased intragastric pressure by nondepolarizing muscle relaxants and lidocaine. Anesthesiology 34:185, 1971.

17. Kosaka Y, Takahashi T, Mark LC: Intrvenous thiobarbiturate anesthesia for cesarean section. Anesthesiology 31:489, 1969.
18. Peltz B, Sinclair DM: Induction agents for cesarean section. A comparison of thiopental and ketamine. Anaesthesia 28:37,

1973.
19. Hodgkinson R, et al: Neonatal neurobehavioral tests following cesarean section under general and spinal anesthesia. Am J Obstet Gynecol 132:67, 1978.
20. Schultetus RR, et al: Ketamine vs. thiopental as induction agents for cesarean section. Anesthesiology A306, 1981.
21. Sellick BA: Cricoid pressure to control regurgitation of stomach contents during induction of anesthesia. Lancet 2:404, 1961.
22. Marx FG, Joshi CW, Orkin LR: Placental transmission of nitrous oxide. Anesthesiology 32:429, 1970.
23. Moir DD: Anesthesia for caesarean section. An evaluation of a method using low concentrations of halothane and 50 per cent of oxygen. Br J Anesth 42:136-142, 1970.
24. Dick W, Knoche E, Traub E: Clinical investigations concerning the use of Ethrane for cesarean section. J Perinat Med 7:125-133, 1979.
25. Andersen T, et al: Cardiovascular effects of rapid intravenous injection of synthetic oxytocin during elective cesarean section. Clin Pharmacol Therapeut 6:345-349, 1965.
26. Scanlon JW, Brown WU, Weiss JB, et al: Neurobehavioral responses of newborn infants after maternal epidural anesthesia. Anesthesiology 40:121-128, 1974.
27. McGuiness JA: Epidural anesthesia with bupivacaine for cesarean section. Anesthesiology 45:270, 1978.
28. Corke BC: Neurobehavioural responses of the newborn. Anaesthesia 32:539-543, 1977.
29. Abboud TK, et al: Maternal, fetal, and neonatal responses after epidural anesthesia with bupivacaine, 2-chloroprocaine, or lidocaine. Anesth Analg 61:638, 1982.
30. Gutsche BB: Prophylactic ephedrine preceding spinal analgesia for cesarean section. Anesthesiology 45:462, 1976.
31. Gibbs CP, Spohr L, Petrakis J, et al: Prevention of hypotension with hydration. Anesthesiology 55:A308, 1981.
32. Caritis SN, Abouleish E, Edelstone DI, et al: Fetal acid-base state following spinal or epidural anesthesia for cesarean section. Obstet Gynecol 56:610, 1980.
33. Kenepp NB, Shelley WC, Kumar S, et al: Effects on newborn of hydration with glucose in patients undergoing cesarean section with regional anesthesia. Lancet 1:654, 1980.
34. Mathru M, et al: Intravenous albumin administration for prevention of spinal hypotension during cesarean section. Anesth Analg 59:655, 1980.
35. Datta S, et al: Acid-base status of diabetic mothers and their infants following spinal anesthesia for cesarean section. Anesth Analg 61:662, 1982.
36. James FM, Greiss FC, Jr, Kemp RA: A comparison of general anesthesia and lumbar epidural analgesia for elective cesarean section. Anesth Analg 56:228, 1976.
37. Datta S, Brown WU: Acid-base status in diabetic mothers and their infants following general or spinal anesthesia for cesarean section. Anesthesiology 47:272, 1977.
38. Shoemaker WC: Crystalloids, colloids, and blood products. ASA Refresher Course 126B, 1981.
39. Ravindran RS, Bond VK, Tasch MD, et al: Prolonged neural blockade following regional analgesia with 2-chloroprocaine.

Anesth Analg 59:447, 1980.
40. Reisner LS, Hochman BN, Plumer MH: Persistent neurologic deficit and adhesive arachnoiditis following intrathecal 2-chloroprocaine injection. Anesth Analg 59:452, 1980.
41. Moore, DC, Spierdijk J, vanKleef JD, et al: Chloroprocaine neurotoxicity: Four additional cases. Anesth Analg 61:155, 1982.
42. Gibbs CP, Munson ES: Local anesthetic toxicity (Letters to the Editor). Anesth Analg 59:955, 1980.
43. Barsa JE, Batra M, Fink RB: Prolonged neural blockade following regional analgesia with 2-chloroprocaine (Letters to the Editor). Anesth Analg 59:810, 1980.
44. Ravindran RS, Turner M, Miller J: Neurological effects of subarachnoid injection of large volumes of 2-chloroprocaine, bupivacaine, and low pH (3.0) saline in dogs. Anesthesiology 55:A163, 1981.
45. Rosen MA, Baysinger CL, Shnider SM, et al: Evaluation of neurotoxicity of local anesthetics following subarachnoid injection. Anesthesiology 57:A196, 1982.
46. Wang BC, Spielholz NI, Hillman DE, et al: Subarachnoid sodium bisulfite (the antioxidant in nesacaine) causes chronic neurological deficit. Anesthesiology 57:A194, 1982.
47. Covino BG, Marx FG, Finster M, et al: Prolonged sensory/ motor following inadvertent spinal anesthesia. Anesth Analg 59:399, 1980.
48. Moore DC, Batra MS: The components of an effective test dose prior to epidural block. Anesthesiology 55:693, 1981.
49. Albright GA: Cardiac arrest following regional anesthesia with etidocaine or bupivacaine (Editorial Views). Anesthesi ology 51:285, 1979.
50. Liu P, Feldman HS, Covino BG: Comprative CNS and cardiovascular toxicity of various local anesthetic agents. Anesthesiology 55:A156, 1981.
51 Avery P, Redon D, Schaenzer G, et al: Cerebral and cardiac toxicity of bupivacaine in the presence of normokalemia versus hyperkalemia. Anesthesiology 55:A164, 1981.
52. Loehning RW, Tanz RD: Bupivacaine ismore cardiotoxic than lidocaine. Anesthesiology 55:A165, 1981.
53. Prentiss JE: Cardiac arrest following caudal anesthesia. Anesthesiology 50:51, 1979.

NEW ASPECTS OF NONDEPOLARIZING RELAXANT REVERSAL

JOHN J. SAVARESE, M.D.

Much of the recent information regarding the clinical pharmacology of nondepolarizing relaxant reversal has been produced by the San Francisco group (Cronnelly, Miller, Fahey, Morris, et al).

Very briefly, neostigmine and pyridostigmine are still the "standard" reversal agents. The San Francisco group has compared the relative potencies and pharmacokinetics of the two standard drugs with edrophonium (Tensilon[R]). Surprisingly, at equipotent dosage (edrophonium 0.5 mg/kg , neostigmine 0.043 mg/kg, pyridostigmine 0.35 mg/kg), the duration of antagonistic effect of edrophonium is equal to that of neostigmine but shorter than that of pyridostigmine. Thus, edrophonium at dosage of 0.5-1.0 mg/kg provides fully effective and sustained antagonism of nondepolarizing block. The measured kinetic parameters (Table 1) support the initial clinical measurements made by Kopman and by Bevan's group (see references).

Table 1 Pharmacokinetic Variables for Anticholinesterase Agents

Drug	Dose	T½α (min)	T½β (min)	Vdss (L/kg)	Cl (ml/kg/min)
edrophonium	0.5mg/kg	7.2	110	1.1	9.6
neostigmine	0.043mg/kg	3.5	80	0.7	9.0
pyridostigmine	0.35mg/kg		112	1.1	8.6

The kinetic parameters show that the pattern and timing of distribution and elimination of edrophonium throughout the body is quite similar to that of neostigmine.

Further studies by the San Francisco group have highlighted the clinical advantages of edrophonium: (A) at 0.5-1.0 mg/kg, edrophonium shows a faster onset of its antagonistic action than neostigmine (3), and (B) edrophonium requires less atropine for prevention of bradycardia than neostigmine, since edrophonium is a much weaker muscarinic stimulant than neostigmine (6). In fact, only 0.7 mg atropine is required to prevent bradycardia secondary to edrophonium 0.5-1.0 mg/kg. For these reasons, edrophonium may represent an advance in the clinical reversal of nondepolarizing block, especially in view of the shorter duration of action of the newer nondepolarizing relaxants.

The San Francisco group has also certainly allayed our fears concerning "recurarization" in patients in renal failure who have received nondepolarizing relaxants. In this group of subjects, elimination of relaxant is 2-5 times slower than in normal subjects. Therefore, if the elimination half-lives of the antagonists were unaffected by renal failure, then it might be expected that the antagonistic effect of the anticholinesterases might be outlasted by the nondepolarizing blocker. Kinetic studies have shown, however, that the half-lives of edrophonium, neostigmine and pyridostigmine are prolonged by renal failure to at least the same degree as the half-lives of the presently available nondepolarizing relaxants. Consequently, the relaxant's effect should not persist longer than the antagonist's effect, even in patients in renal failure (ref 1,2,4). The new nondepolarizing relaxants, which rely much less on the kidney for their elimination, will lead to much more facile handling of nondepolarizing block and its antagonism in these patients.

REFERENCES

1. Cronnelly R, Stanski DR, Miller RD, et al: Renal function and the pharmacokinetics of neostigmine in anesthetized man. Anesthesiology 51:222, 1979.
2. Cronnelly R, Stanski DR, Miller RD, et al: Pyridostigmine kinetics with and without renal function. Clin Pharmacol Ther 28:78, 1980.
3. Morris R, Cronnelly R, Miller RD, et al: Pharmacokinetics of edrophonium and neostigmine when antagonizing d-tubocurarine neuromuscular blockade in man. Anesthesiology 54:399, 1981.
4. Morris R, Cronnelly R, Miller RD, et al: Pharmacokinetics of edrophonium in anephric and renal transplant patients. Brit J Anaesth 53:1311, 1981.
5. CronnellyR, Morris R: Antagonism of neuromuscular blockade. Brit J Anaesth 54:183, 1982.

6. Cronnelly R, Morris R, Miller RD: Edrophonium: Duration of action and atropine requirement in man during halothane anesthesia. Anesthesiology 1982.
7. Kopman A: Edrophonium antagonism of pancuronium-induced neuromuscular blockade in man: a reappraisal. Anesthesiology 51:139, 1979.
8. Beavan DR: Reversal of pancuronium with edrophonium. Anaesthesia 34:614-619, 1979.

BUYING A MONITOR

N. TY SMITH, M.D.

Buying a monitor can be one of the most difficult tasks in all of anesthesia. To decide whether to use a new drug is relatively easy and usually requires only a slight to moderate adjustment of one's thinking. Monitoring, on the other hand, can be a whole new world: 1) The purchase, use, and maintenance of monitoring equipment can constitute a major budget item. 2) Extensive physical modifications may be be required for the operating rooms and the operating suite. 3) Hazards to the user, as well as the patient, may exist. 4) To use and to interpret these devices often require new and technical knowledge. 5) This knowledge is usually not taught in medical school or in residency programs.

A short presentation cannot dispel all of these difficulties, nor for that matter, can an entire course. Unfortunately, neither can most articles or books on the subject. We can, however, examine a few practical approaches to some of these problems. You can then apply this type of thinking to your problems in monitoring. The questions we shall approach are based on three literature references which were selected not for their relationship to each other, but rather because they illustrate well some of the problems involved in buying a monitor. 1) How do you decide that you need a monitor?1 2) How do you select a monitor in general?2 3) As an example, how do you select an oxygen monitor?3

1. <u>Preventable anesthesia mishaps: A study of human factors1.</u>

Perhaps the best way to decide whether one needs a

monitor is to consult the series of papers coming from the Massachusetts General Hospital. We shall examine one which appeared in _Anesthesiology_[1]. This describes a survey of "critical incidents", that is, anesthetic accidents or near accidents occurring in the operating room. Essentially, the authors are using the same techniques as those used in airplane accidents to try to determine the incidence, type and cause of anesthetic misadventures. In this and subsequent surveys, the authors concluded that most of the accidents were "pilot error," and that the cause often related to human factors, such as distraction, fatigue, irritation or boredom. Good monitoring can improve this situation; poor monitoring could make it worse. Some of the more common accidents which were emphasized in this paper and which could be dealt with by monitoring are 1) airway disconnects, 2) problems with the anesthesia machine, and 3) gas supply problems.

The first problem, airway disconnects, can be dealt with in several ways: continuous observation of and contact with the patient, an esophageal or conventional stethoscope, continuous airway pressure recordings, or electrical disconnect alarms. Each of these has its problems, and none is fool-proof yet. They demonstrate that no matter what the monitor, there is no substitute for continuous observation and thinking.

The second problem, the anesthesia machine, can be dealt with with a simple monitoring technique -- a check list to be checked before _each_ case. This requires nothing more than a sheet of paper and some time, and can save considerable grief.

The third set of problems, those related to gas supply, can best be attacked with an inspired-gas oxygen monitor. Choosing an oxygen monitor will be discussed later. Suffice it to say, an inspired oxygen tension monitor is the _only_ final common pathway to solving all these immediately hazardous problems of gas supply.

2. _Selection of monitoring equipment_[2].

Choosing a monitor can be frustrating and time consuming. It is tempting to hand the task over to the hospital's biomedical engineer, if you are fortunate enough to have one. On the other hand, it is you, not he, who has to live with the monitor and depend on it on a daily basis. Therefore, the more active you are in its choice, the better. One does not have to have an exensive technical background to avoid some of the worst pitfalls in selecting a monitor. A chapter by Nobel and Kostinsky2 describes in detail the selection of a monitor. I would like to summarize some of their points and to add a few of my own.

1) Select <u>one</u> manufacturer for all of the monitoring equipment in the hospital. It will make in-hospital service and repair easier.

2) Do not necessarily buy the cheapest. It may be the most expensive to operate.

3) Approach the first production units with caution. Someone has to buy the first unit, but it does not have to be you.

4) Seek the opinion of others. You frequently seek opinions from your colleagues in medical situations. Do the same with the expensive equipment you purchase. The best advice may come from someone who already owns and uses the equipment you are considering.

5) Check out the equipment at delivery. It is reported that up to 40-50% of monitoring equipment is defective in some way. Get it fixed before you start using it.

6) Require a performance and safety check as a condition for sale. Do not establish that it is unsafe after the equipment is installed and about to be used -- or already being used.

7) Have an extensive training program for everyone who will be using the equipment. A good monitoring equipment company will help you set up a program.

8) If you cannot maintain it, do not buy it. It will not operate forever without a certain amount of care and

repair.

9) Check out the controls. For example, are they few in number, conveniently located, clearly labeled and easy to use?

10) Be careful with alarms. Those fancy alarms may look good during a demonstration, but may become a frustration because they are influenced too frequently by artifacts or other sometimes uncontrollable circumstances.

3. Oxygen monitoring and end-tidal gas analysis in anesthesia.3

An inspired oxygen monitor may be one of the first devices which you will choose, after an anesthesia machine.3 The importance of having an oxygen monitor on anesthesia machines cannot be over-emphasized. An oxygen monitor can save lives, save money, and help prevent pollution; there is no substitute for in-line oxygen analysis. To my knowledge, it is the only monitor which can be proved to be effective both in saving lives and saving money. The 10 principles listed above apply to the purchase of any monitor, including an oxygen monitor. The subsequent list describes some of the problems especially prominent with oxygen monitors, although they can obviously apply to other monitors.

1) Choose a reputable manufacturer which has a representative who is readily accessible and who understands the instrument.

2) Determine how and by whom preventive maintenance procedures will be performed. These devices typically require more frequent service than other anesthesia apparatus. Some are easier to service than others. Is your practice set up to assure that the maintenance will be performed at necessary intervals? If not, you will probably decide that oxygen monitors are "unreliable." It takes very little training to maintain some of these devices, and some departments maintain their own oxygen monitors.

3) The relative merits of power from a replaceable

battery, a rechargeable battery vs only the ac line should be considered. If there is an ac line very close to the machine, then it is certainly the most convenient source, since it eliminates all worry about batteries running out. On the other hand, if the AC outlet is far away, the power cable may become a potential trip-line. Rechargeable batteries represent a good compromise: they can be charged at night when no one is around. A nonexplosive unit is most likely to be battery-powered.

4) There are two major types of sensors: fuel cell and polarographic. The major advantage of the fuel cell for anesthetists is that is is not sensitive to nitrous oxide. On the other hand, the polarographic sensor is consumed only when it is turned on; the fuel cell, by definition, is continuously being burned up when it is exposed to any oxygen.

5) Compute the true operating cost by estimating the cost of maintenance in addition to instrument purchase price. Sensor replacement and servicing can be a significant expense, exceeding within two years the purchase price of the instrument. Closely examine the manufacturer's estimate of the life of the sensor, the warranty, and the replacement costs. Buying oxygen monitors is analagous to buying razors; you might purchase an inexpensive razor for which you must buy expensive blades for the rest of your life. This is the area where bargaining with several manufacturers for an advantageous warranty or sensor-replacement contract is crucial.

6) Decide how much time you are willing to devote to calibrating the instrument at the start of each procedure. The longer the instrument's response time, the longer you will have to wait for it to stabilize for calibration. (Polarographic sensors are typically faster than fuel-cell sensors.)

7) Inspect the alarm characteristics. Some alarms can be accidentally deactivated -- for example, set to 0% O2 -- and may not help when most needed. An alarm that can be

temporarily silenced can avoid some aggravation.

8) If you will want to sterilize the sensor after it has been exposed to a contaminated atmosphere, check with the manufacturer to find out if it can be done. Try it out yourself.

9) None of the models are affected by "humidity", but some may be affected if excessive condensate forms on the sensor. This is likely to happen on the expired side of a breathing circuit or in low-flow applications.

10) Evaluate the monitor in the presence of an operating electro-surgical unit.

11) Determine if the monitor can be mounted in an accessible location within your present system.

12) Do not purchase a monitor until you have actually used it for a while (at least 30 days) to see how well it will fit into your routine and how well it performs under actual operating room conditions.

13) Make sure that a fitting or connector is available to connect the sensor to the anesthesia machine.

14) Some units are not to be used in explosive atmospheres; this may or may not be important to you.

HOW TO DECIDE IF A MONITOR FITS YOUR NEEDS

In this part our discussion, I am going to be the devil's advocate. The basic thesis will be that the same enthusiasm and excitement for a new technology brought forth by a manufacturer may not be matched by the ultimate user in the operating room. My complaint is that wonderful devices based on brilliant insight into sound physical/engineering principles are often generated without consulting the ultimate user, who could help plan in a detailed way every feature of the device. So often the manufacturer gives the anesthetist an answer in search of a question. It may be better for those creating new technologies to look for clinical problems that need solving; this could be accomplished on a continuing basis by questioning those who are involved with these problems daily.

Why do some monitoring devices survive and others fall by the wayside? Perhaps we can obtain a partial answer by using the operating room as a microcosm of the overall problem. I shall focus on a list of criteria for acceptance of a cardiovascular monitor in the operating room. The list is meant to be neither complete nor absolute. On the other hand, it could be useful in helping you decide whether a new device or monitor will be useful to you. Or perhaps the list can help compare different types of technology or different monitors.

Table 1 outlines 21 technologically achievable criteria for cardiovascular monitors in the operating room. Many of these criteria are self-evident. Others may require some explanation. For the remainder of this section, I shall give the number of a criterion and a brief explanation if appropriate. Although all of this section is devoted to the cardiovascular system, the thought processes involved can be transferred to any monitor or monitoring system for the operating room. A somewhat different set of criteria would have to be used for the intensive care unit.

TABLE ONE

TWENTY-SEVEN TECHNOLOGICALLY ATTAINABLE CRITERIA FOR

EVALUATING CARDIOVASCULAR MONITORS

1) Measures a function of the CVS, as directly as possible.
2) Small in size.
3) Fits into OR (size, shape, color....).
4) Easy to clean.
5) Quiet (silent).
6) Indestructible.
7) Inexpensive.

8) Compatible with other OR devices, especially electronically.
9) Electrically safe.
10) No side effects from long-term monitoring.
11) No pain or discomfort to patient (noninvasive).
12) Easy and rapid application of transducer or sensor.
13) Easy and rapid calibration.
14) Works on all patients at all times.
15) Reproducible results when taken off patient and reapplied by different people and/or on different days.
16) Stable and reliable for several hours - transducer may be inaccessible during surgery.
17) Insensitive to movement of transducer.
18) Insensitive to movement of connecting lines or cables.
19) Impervious to electrocautery.
20) No disturbance of surgery.
21) No disturbance by surgeon or surgical procedure.
22) Easily read output, with some meaning to anesthetist.
23) Output continuous, preferably with a trend recorder.
24) Early warning from the output, that is, before rapid deterioration or irreversibility sets in.
25) Low incidence of false positives, and negatives, that is, ability to separate a routine depression from one signalling danger.
26) Should be clear that when it has failed, it has failed.
27) Something really needed by anesthetists.

The following is an elaboration of some of the points briefly outlined in the table.

1. A function of the cardiovascular system would relate, for example, to pressure, contractility, output of the heart, or heart rate. A direct measurement would be the

measurement of pressure through an arterial cannula. An indirect measurement would be estimating the sizeof the heart by ultrasound. Direct measurements are theoretically better; indirect measurements are far more practical for monitoring.

4. Monitors seem to attract dust, especially in any hard to clean corners. In addition, dirt and germs seem to have a mutual attraction.

5. The operating room is a noisy enough place.

6. The operating room is a hostile environment at best. All efforts seem to be directed at destroying equipment.

9. If the OR is mechanically hostile, electrically, it is a catastrophe.

10. Side effects may not be easily anticipated simply from examining the technology. For example, the automatic noninvasive blood pressure cuff has many potential problems, such as pooling of drugs, venous congestion, nerve damage, and the inability to measure blood pressure as frequently as may be desired. Furthermore, what may be safe in a healthy individual may be dangerous in a very sick patient.

12. Time is of the essence in the operating room. Five minutes spent in setting up a monitor may not seem like much to the salesman. However, many hospitals charge $600 per hour to the patient for operating room time. If five minutes is multiplied by the approximately 25 million operations per year in the United States, one can see that a considerable amount of time and money is involved. Besides, waiting patiently is not one of our virtues.

14. Some cynics have claimed that the conventional manual method for measuring blood pressure (cuff and stethoscope) works well unless a patient is in shock, is undergoing therapy to increase blood pressure, is hypothermic, or when the blood pressure is very low. In other words, the method works except at the times when it is really needed.

15. People of all stages of training, ability, attentiveness, or reliability may use the technology. In other words, the technology must not only be foolproof, it

must be anesthetist proof. A manufacturer could argue, "Why not hire a technician to run my device?" Unfortunately, that adds cost to the use of the device, and the extra person in the operating room may increase the risk of infection or distraction.

16. Thus a transducer which is close to the patient and which requires constant attention, manipulation, or readjustment is simply worthless in the operating room, because of the constraints of sterile fields and drapes and aseptic personnel.

17. If a technology involves a microphone placed on the chest, for example,and the surgeons insist on throwing their instruments onto the chest, there may be some problems.

18. The slightest movement of the catheter connecting the arterial line to the transducer will produce gross artifact in the blood pressure measurement. This is obviously an intolerable situation, which we still tolerate.

19. Probably the single biggest curse of the operating room is the electrocautery. Up to 5,000 volts may be applied. The current goes through the patient and out a grounding point; and patient, air, and electrical circuits are filled with white electrical noise. In addition, if grounding paths are not correct, the electrocautery can produce burns in the patient, often serious.

20. If the monitor requires an electrode on the chest and the surgeon wishes to operate on the chest, try to imagine who will win that battle.

21. One of the earliest and best examples of this problem is the surgeon who insists on continually bumping the blood pressure cuff, producing sounds which imitate those trying to be interpreted either by the human ear or by a machine. In this particular instance,the human ear does better than the machine, but even then it may be a problem to measure the correct blood pressure.

22. The anesthetist has often been described as a one-arm paper hanger on roller skates. He is, or should be, continually scanning the patient, the operation, the

anesthesia machine, the infusion of drugs, and the administration of the anesthetic. He should not be required to devote too much attention too long at a time to any one area.

23. Since events can occur very rapidly in the operating room, a monitor that produces an output every 30 minutes or an hour, for example, would not be able to produce information rapidly enough. A continuous trend recorder helps spot difficulties often long before absolute values might.

24. We have little use for a monitor that tells us that the patient has just died.

25. If there are too many false positives, the user will not use the monitor, because it becomes too bothersome. If there are too many false negatives, the user will not trust the monitor. Obviously, some compromise has to be made, and certainly in this instance, there must be education on the part of the physician as well as on the part of the developers of monitors.

26. The use of computers in monitoring equipment sometimes changes the original information so much that it is impossible to tell, for example, whether artifact is occurring.

27. This bring us in a full circle to the original point of this section; the technology must be developed for the user, not for the creator.

REFERENCES

1. Cooper JB, Newbower RS, Long CD, McPeek B: Preventable anesthesia mishaps: A study of human factors. Anesthesiology 49: 399-406, 1978.

2. Nobel J, Kostinsky H: Selection of monitoring equipment. In LJ Saidman and N Ty Smith (Eds), Monitoring in Anesthesia, Wiley and Sons, Inc., New York, 1978, pp. 261-282.

3. Smith N Ty, Rader CD: Oxygen monitoring and end-tidal gas analysis in anesthesia. Cardiovascular Pulmonary Technology, August/September, 1977.

WHEN ARE PULMONARY ARTERY CATHETERS INDICATED IN NONCARDIAC SURGERY?

CASEY D. BLITT, M.D.

The flow-guided pulmonary artery catheter (Swan-Ganz) represents a major advance in the clinician's ability to evaluate cardiac performance. This catheter permits measurement of cardiac output, calculation of systemic and pulmonary vascular resistances, and mixed venous blood can be obtained for calculation of intrapulmonary shunt. Newer catheters even permit cardiac pacing to be performed with one of these catheters.

Certain groups of patients can benefit from a pulmonary artery catheter. Indications for pulmonary artery catheters in noncardiac surgery are not etched in stone by any means, but clinical experience over the last five to seven years has ferreted out certain subgroups of patients whose perioperative management can be improved with a pulmonary artery catheter.

One group of patients that can benefit from a pulmonary artery catheter are those with pre-existing moderate to severe cardiac disease. The question always arises, "What is moderate to severe cardiac disease?" The following criteria can help identify a patient with significant cardiac disease. Any of the following criteria are indications for insertion of a pulmonary artery catheter:

1. Goldman Risk Class III or greater (13 points or more)
2. LVEDP greater than 20 mmHg
3. Ejection fraction less than 50%
4. Recent or poorly controlled congestive heart failure
5. Angiographically confirmed coronary artery disease
6. Recent myocardial infarction
7. Noncompliant left ventricle, aortic stenosis, hypertrophic cardiomyopathies

Some of these criteria depend upon information gleaned as a result of cardiac catheterization or coronary angiography and frequently this information is not always available. As noninvasive cardiac diagnostic modalities become perfected, we will have this information more frequently.

Moderate to severe pulmonary disease can also be defined by using certain criteria. These criteria are as follows:

1. FEV/FVC less than 60%
2. Poor preoperative oxygenation (PO_2 less than 55 on room air)
3. MVV less than 50% of predicted
4. Predicted need for PEEP
5. Interstitial edema on chest x-ray

Should patients with moderate to severe cardiac or pulmonary disease receive a pulmonary artery catheter if the operation is relatively minor? Certainly, the need for a pulmonary artery catheter is somewhat dependent upon the surgical procedure. Major surgical procedures such as thoracotomies, bowel resections, and extensive cancer surgery would be more of an indication for a pulmonary artery catheter in these patients than excision of a ganglion. Patients who are anticipated to have marked shifts in fluids and marked requirements for volume replacement (with cardiac or pulmonary disease) should be considered candidates for a pulmonary artery catheter.

Our ASA Physical Status classification may be of some help to us in deciding who needs a pulmonary artery catheter. Patients classified ASA III or greater may benefit from a pulmonary artery catheter. To amplify on an item listed under Cardiac Disease (myocardial infarction), I would like to review a study by Rao and his colleagues. They looked at myocardial reinfarction following anesthesia in patients who had a recent myocardial infarction. It is well known that myocardial reinfarction following anesthesia and surgery is very high in patients who have an infarct less than 6 months old. Dr. Rao and his colleagues anesthetized 97 patients over a 3-year period who had a documented myocardial infarction that was less than 6 months old. The patients were divided into those whose infarcts were less than 3 months old and those whose infarcts were between 3 and 6 months old. Pulmonary artery catheters and arterial lines were inserted in all of these patients prior to induction of anesthesia and the patients were continuously monitored during the operative procedure and in the postoperative period. Appropriate measures were taken to prevent deleterious cardiovascular reflexes during laryngoscopy and intubation and throughout the anesthetic course hemodynamic and vascular volume status were carefully controlled. Utilizing this regimen, the authors were able to decrease the reinfarction rate and mortality dramatically. As a result of this study, I would recommend that a recent myocardial infarction and emergency or required surgery necessitates a pulmonary artery catheter. It has also been shown that pulmonary capillary wedge pressure may show myocardial ischemia before ST segment changes.

A large group of patients who have been shown to benefit from a PA catheter are those undergoing vascular operations where aortic cross-clamping and unclamping is anticipated. The information obtained from PA catheterization is crucial to titrate volume, vasodilators or vasopressors for optimal control of each patient's hemodynamic status during operations where the aorta is cross-clamped.

Another group of patients recently shown to benefit from a pulmonary artery catheter are neurosurgical patients. Craniotomies performed in the sitting position or other neurosurgical procedures where air embolism is a consideration represent an indication for pulmonary artery catheterization. The pulmonary artery catheter helps us decide what air emboli are significant and also tells us when the effect of the air embolism has subsided. The pulmonary artery pressure rises substantially during air embolus and its return to baseline values tells us that the physiologic insult is over. The pulmonary artery catheter has been shown to correlate well with end tidal carbon dioxide. Recent evidence has also shown that right atrial pressure may be greater than left atrial pressure in the sitting position. It is helpful to know when this condition occurs because this situation could predispose to paradoxical embolism. It is my recommendation that a pulmonary artery catheter should be considered a valuable monitoring device in sitting neurosurgical procedures to be used along with a Doppler and end tidal carbon dioxide. In this same regard, the pulmonary artery catheter is valuable in barbiturate coma so as to keep preload adequate so that cardiac depression does not occur as a result of administration of large doses of barbiturate.

The ability of the pulmonary artery catheter balloon to manipulate pulmonary blood flow has been recently investigated. Pulmonary blood flow can be manipulated to divert blood away from a nonventilated lung. Thus, pulmonary artery balloon manipulation of blood flow may be of value in treating severe unilateral lung disease with systemic hypoxemia. From a clinical standpoint, this might be useful in thoracic surgery to shift blood from the upper lung to the lower lung in thoracic surgery.

References

1. Rao TK, El-Etr AA: Myocardial reinfarction following anesthesia in patients with recent infarction. (Personal Communication)

2. Marshall WK, Bedford RF: Use of a pulmonary artery catheter for detection and treatment of venous air embolism. Anesthesiology 52:131-134, 1980.

3. Alfery DD, Zamost BG, Benumof JL: Unilateral lung lavage: blood flow manipulation by ipsilateral pulmonary artery balloon inflation in dogs. Anesthesiology 55:376-380, 1981.

4. Silverstein PR, Caldera DL, Cullen DJ: Avoiding the hemodynamic consequences of aortic cross-clamping and unclamping. Anesthesiology 50:462-466, 1979.

5. Lunn JK, Dannemiller FJ, Stanley TH: Cardiovascular responses to clamping of the aorta during epidural and general anesthesia. Anesthesia & Analgesia (Cleve) 58:372-376, 1979.

6. Kaplan JA, Wells PH: Early diagnosis of myocardial ischemia using the pulmonary artery catheter. Anesthesia & Analgesia (Cleve) 60:789-793, 1981.

7. DelGuercio LRM, Cohn JD: Monitoring operative risk in the elderly. JAMA 243:1350-1355, 1980.

8. Perkins-Pearson NAK, Marshall WK, Bedford RF: Atrial pressures and air embolism in the seated position. Anesthesiology 55:A236, 1981.

MONITORING THE EEG IN THE OPERATING ROOM

N. TY SMITH, M.D.

The EEG was the first electronic monitor to be used in the operating room. It has undergone periods of enthusiasm and disillusionment during its nearly 40-year career. There are several reasons for the problems and the lack of enthusiasm which the EEG has encountered 1. First, unlike the ECG, it is a difficult wave form to interpret unless one has had considerable training. Although some EEG patterns are easy to interpret, such as enflurane seizures, most are not for the average neurological layman. Another problem involves the way the EEG is conventionally displayed - either on a fairly rapidly moving strip chart or on an oscilloscope screen. With the former, a permanent record is achieved, but at the cost of a very large amount of paper - generated at a rate of 300 pages an hour. It is extremely difficult to shuffle through these pages and compare what is happening presently to the patient with what happened during induction or three hours ago, for example. An oscilloscope is no better. Although it does not waste paper, it only provides a fleeting display, which must be remembered and compared with previous patterns in one's own mind. In its present state of affairs, the EEG is not easy to set up, and requires a trained technician to apply electrodes properly. This is in definite contrast to the ECG; whose electrode technology is currently so advanced that even an anesthesiologist can properly apply the electrodes. The EEG is a much lower voltage than the ECG, about 10-30 times, and consequently is even more sensitive to electrical or mechanical noise which so often occurs in the operating room. A partial solution to the problem could be not only to hire a technician, but to hire an experienced interpreter of the EEG to constantly be in the operating room and provide information on the status of the EEG to the anesthesiologist. Good EEG interpreters, however, are rare and expensive. What is really needed is a method of displaying the EEG so clearly that the anesthetist can easily interpret it and quickly make intelligent decisions based on his observations. The display should be compressed, so that several minutes or hours of the EEG are presented in a relatively small space.

Twelve years ago we used a computer averaging technique to investigate the EEG in dogs 2. This technique averaged the EEG over, for example, a minute. This spectrum could clearly reflect changes in depth of anesthesia as halothane concentration was increased. If we selected certain parts of the spectrum, such as the sum of two and three Hz, we observed a linear relationship between anesthetic concentration and the EEG. This was also a dynamic relationship, that it, we could change the concentration of halothane and observe a change in the EEG numbers.

About the same time, the so-called Cerebral Function Monitor was being developed in Britain 3. This simple device heavily filters the EEG and presents the resultant EEG in a very compressed form. It was certainly an easy display to interpret: if it went up, that was good; if it went down, that was bad. On the other hand, quite often only gross changes could be detected. Furthermore, changes resulting from changes in anesthetic depth were not consistent. The usefulness of the CFM was demonstrated mainly in catastrophic situations such as cardiac arrest; as a device which followed the frequency of occurrence of seizures, and hence the response to therapy; and most usefully as a device which could follow, again in a compressed fashion, the EEG in a patient suspected of brain death.

A much more sophisticated analysis and display method, the compressed spectral array (CSA), was developed by Bimar in France, expanded at Stanford University, and considerably refined by Bickford 4. The CSA uses a Fourier transform method to produce a spectrum, similar to the one we had produced earlier with a computer of average transients (CAT). Any time period (epoch) can be selected to generate this spectrum. Typically, an epoch is four or eight seconds. The spectrum is then smoothed, and the tracing repeated every four seconds to produce a mountain and valley effect. The result is an easily read three-dimensional display which can pack a considerable amount of information onto a small space. The effects produced by an injection of an anesthetic agent, for example thiopental, is dramatic, and easily detected and read even by the untrained anesthetist. The CSA does have several disadvantages, however. One of the more important is that the mountains if too high often hide information behind them. For this and other reasons we developed the DSA, the density modulated spectral array 5, 6. This works by creating a voice print-like shaded light and dark pattern, achieved by moving a pen across a thermal strip chart recorder. The DSA emphasizes patterns. One can easily see for example the difference between an awake patient and one anesthetized by halothane. Furthermore, each anesthetic agent seems to have its own signature, so that it is easy to tell which anesthetic is being given - if you happen to forget.

Still another technique is the zero-crossing technique, which simply counts the number of times that the EEG crosses a zero line during a specified period of time. This method has been used extensively at Duke University by Klein and Davis. It has been tested with several agents, and is a very easily read display.

The most advanced technique is an aperiodic technique developed by Demetrescu 4. The Demetrescu method detects individual wave forms and plots them on a screen according to frequency, amplitude, (plotted as the height of a "telephone pole"), and time, which appears to move back into the screen. This method preserves the most information of all the methods. Its patterns are often the easiest to detect and to diagnose. On the other hand, because it does preserve so much information, it is not as compact as the display generated by most of the other techniques. Recently the display has been color coded for easier interpretation.

We shall demonstrate these methods during the lecture by examining the effects of a commonly used anesthetic agent, halothane. In general with all of these techniques, halothane produces a band which shifts to the left, that is, decreases in frequency, as concentration increases. This is true with the CSA and the DSA in particular. It therefore seemed appropriate to derive a number which could reflect the depth of anesthesia with halothane, much as we had done with the earlier CAT technique. One of the resulting numbers is the peak power frequency, the frequency which occurs most often in a given period of time. The peak power frequency is related to the concentration of halothane anesthesia, as well as to the tension of CO2 and the period of time over which halothane has been given. Similarly useful is the median power frequency, the frequency which divides the spectrum into two equal areas.

Except for our earlier CAT studies, all of these measurements were taken at steady state-levels. We are also interested to see if the EEG can follow rapidly changing concentrations of anesthetic, since changing depth is a frequent part of anesthetic management. We tested this in several ways. First, we slowly or rapidly changed the concentration of inspired halothane in a sinusoidal fashion. This produced a spectacular display of sinusoidally changing EEG's, both in the CSA and DSA, as well as the MPF. If we gave a brief pulse (or "bolus") of halothane, as short as two minutes, this was reflected very rapidly in the EEG.

Ira Rampil has developed another number derived from the EEG -the spectral edge frequency 7. Again, the spectral edge frequency follows changes in concentration of halothane in a linear fashion. A more difficult problem, as far as EEG display techniques are concerned, is enflurane. The spike-wave activity can contaminate many displays and make some of the numbers difficult to obtain. This is particularly true with the spectral edge frequency. Rampil has developed a "de-spiking technique" which makes the EEG easier to analyze. One of the important and interesting features of the EEG with enflurane is that it is much easier to display in the presence of nitrous oxide than with oxygen alone.

We used the SEF to follow extremely rapidly changing concentrations of halothane and enflurane, including those where the anesthetic was shut off and on as frequently as every twelve seconds 8. With halothane, these rapid changes were somewhat damped, but with enflurane, even brief changes were detected with the EEG. This led us to the conclusion that the EEG is very useful for detecting rapid changes in anesthetic depth. We were also able to see the uptake and elimination of rapidly acting intravenous agents, such as thiopental. Most importantly, because of the automatic gain control feature, the SEF was able to detect very light depths of anesthesia with enflurane.

The aperiodic technique seems to show more detail in its patterns during anesthesia, including inhalation agents halothane and enflurane. Thus, with halothane the band may spread out, while with enflurane, there may be a "carpet" at lighter depths which shifts to a pair of bands at deeper concentrations.

Muscle tremor influences all techniques, unfortunately, but its presence is easiest to detect with the aperiodic analysis technique and with the Klein technique. The latter uses this signal to estimate the adequacy of neuromuscular blockade. There is another use for this otherwise bothersome noise. The onset of muscle tremor often precedes an increase in blood pressure and heart rate in open-heart patients during cannulation procedures. If this change in the EEG is detected soon enough, the cardiovascular stimulation can be prevented by reassurance of the patient or by administration of a small amount of a narcotic or tranquilizer.

The aperiodic technique seems to have its greatest

advantage during anesthesia with narcotic agents, particularly high-dose techniques. Most other EEG methods are simply overwhelmed by the very high amplitude, very low frequency EEG which is characteristic of most narcotics. The Demetrescu technique, however, preserves enough information that changes can be seen even at very deep levels. Using this technique, we have divided the EEG into five classifications, from awake and sedated, to "too deep". These arbitrary patterns correlate well with the actual clinical state, including subsequent cardiovascular changes following stimulating events, such as endotracheal intubation or surgical incision. Thus, over 90% of the time, we are able to predict the likelihood of no, mild, moderate, or marked cardiovascular response to the stimulating event 9.

Many other events and artifacts can confound interpretation of the EEG. These include CO2 and body temperature. Below 30C the EEG changes markedly, decreasing in amplitude and shifting far to the left. In addition, other artifacts, such as a cardiac pacemaker, bumping the leads, 60 Hz noise, and of course the ubiquitous electrocautery, can either alter or destroy the EEG. The analytic techniques differ in their ability to either detect or suppress the presence of artifact.

Although estimation of the depth of anesthesia is an important function of the EEG, many feel that the greatest use of the EEG will come in the early detection of cerebral ischemia. The EEG is particularly suited to this task and can detect cerebral ischemia in the presence of any anesthetic agent - provided that an excess is not given - or even in the presence of hypothermia. (The major exception to this rule is isoflurane, which can produce a silent EEG at clinical concentrations 10. Major episodes of ischemia, those most likely to produce major neurological deficits, such as stroke or coma, can be detected by almost any analytic technique. An example of a particularly valuable use of the EEG is during arterial hypotension. The EEG can probably indicate whether the blood pressure is too low to allow adequate cerebral perfusion and hence whether further therapy is necessary. Sometimes therapy can be more dangerous than the hypotension, and we wish to avoid it if possible.

Another obvious, and extremely useful, area for the EEG is carotid endarterectomy surgery. The decision on the adequacy of blood pressure, whether to use a shunt or not, the effects of clamping, and the effects of release of shunt, can all be seen with the EEG. Rampil et al 11 observed over 100 patients during endarterectomy surgery, and have seen no false negatives or no false positives in the prediction of postoperative neurologic sequelae, provided that the patient was neurologically normal before surgery.

The EEG is also very useful in open-heart surgery. Adequacy of pump perfusion pressure, detection of problems with the bypass machine, and the presence of emboli can all be detected by the EEG under appropriate conditions. So many different events can influence the EEG during open-heart surgery, however, that interpretation is not as easy as, for example, with carotid endarterectomy surgery. However, if the pump is turned off, we are able to decide when it should be turned on again, even during hypothermia. We have even detected EEG changes occasionally during lifting of the heart and resultant hypotension.

Although we have concentrated mainly on patients undergoing open-heart or carotid surgery, we have occasionally monitored other patients and have been surprised at the number of EEG hypoxic changes. One occurred when a ventilator was shut off for 30 seconds in an abdominal-vascular case. The other occurred during a routine period of apnea during reversal of a neuromuscular block, while allowing CO_2 to accumulate. Apparently the patient was becoming hypoxic, as evidenced by the EEG. Although we do not currently routinely use EEG monitoring other than during open-heart surgery, carotid endarterectomies or deliberate hypotension, perhaps we should use the EEG more routinely than we do presently.

In summary, the EEG has much to offer the anesthetist. Unfortunately, it is still in its infancy. Many problems remain to be solved. We still do not have a good way of placing electrodes or recording the EEG; nor do we have the necessary experience to determine when it is useful and when it is indicated. We also do not have an insight as to which displays are the most useful. Unfortunately, there are so many displays now, that the situation has become very difficult. I suspect that each display has strong points and weak points. For example, the DSA is better with halothane, while the Demetrescu technique is better with high-dose narcotic anesthesia. It may well be that only a technique which retains a considerable amount of information during processing, such as the Demestrescu technique, will ultimately prove to be versatile enough to be used in all cases.

Only time and work will tell.

References:

1. Smith, N Ty: Monitoring the electroencephalogram in the operating room, in Monitoring Surgical Patients in the Operating Room, Gravenstein JS, Newbower RS, Ream AK, Smith N Ty (Eds.), Charles C Thomas, Springfield, Illinois, 1979, pp. 119-141.

2. Lopes da Silva FH, Smith, N Ty, Zwart A and Nichols WW: Spectral analysis of the EEG during halothane anesthesia. Input-output relations. Electroenceph Clin Neurophysiol 33: 311-319, Sept 1972.

3. Prior PF: Monitoring Cerebral Function, JP Lippincott Company, Philadelphia, Pennsylvania, 1979, 360 pp.

4. Smith N Ty: Computers in anesthesia. In LJ Saidman and N Ty Smith (Eds), Monitoring in Anesthesia, Wiley and Sons, Inc., New

York, 1978, pp. 283-329.

5. Fleming RA, Smith N Ty: Density modulation: A technique for the display of three-variable data in patient monitoring, Anesthesiology 50: 543-546, 1979.

6. Fleming RA, Smith N Ty: An inexpensive device for analyzing and monitoring the electroencephalogram, Anesthesiology 50: 456-460, 1979.

7. Rampil IF, Sasse FJ, Smith N Ty et al: Spectral Edge Frequency - A New Correlate of Anesthetic Depth (Abstract), Anesthesiology 53: 3S, pp. S12, 1980.

8. Smith N Ty, Rampil IJ, Sasse FJ, Hoff BH, Flemming DC: EEG during rapidly changing halothane or enflurane. Anesthesiology 51: S4, 1979.

9. Smith N Ty, Demetrescu M: The EEG During High-Dose Fentanyl Anesthesia (Abstract), Anesthesiology 553: 3S, pp. S7, 1980.

10. Eger, II, EI: Monitoring the Depth of Anesthesia. In L Saidman and N Ty Smith _Monitoring in Anesthesia_, John Wiley & Sons, New York, 1978, pp.1-14.

11. Rampil IJ, Holzer JA, Correll JW, Smith N Ty: Prognostic value of computerized EEG monitoring during cerebro-vascular surgery (Abstract), Anesthesiology 55: A126, 1981.

BIOCHEMICAL AND BIOPHYSICAL MONITORING OF THE FETUS

M. FINSTER, M.D.

The ability to determine fetal well-being during or even before labor is an important requirement if fetal and neonatal wastage is to be prevented. Until recently, the physician caring for the pregnant woman had to rely on rather primitive and grossly inaccurate modalities of fetal surveillance, namely, palpation of the abdomen, observation of the character of the amniotic fluid and intermittent auscultation of the fetal heart. Newer methods, introduced in the last 20 years, are based on advanced biophysical and biochemical technology and allow for greater accuracy in monitoring. Their understanding is mandatory for all physicians who participate in the care of the mother and her offspring.

Assessment of the acid-base state of the fetus during labor first became possible in the early 1960's with the development by Saling of a fetal capillary blood-sampling technique. Blood is usually obtained from the scalp but may equally well be collected from the buttocks in a breech presentation. The patient is placed in the lithotomy position, and a conical endoscope is introduced into the vagina. With a light source attached, the endoscope is advanced through the cervix and applied against the skin of the fetus. The skin is dried with cotton swabs and covered with a thin layer of silicone jel in order to minimize the adhesive forces of the surface and facilitate globule formation by the blood sample. A puncture incision is made with a guarded blade and the drop of blood which appears is collected into heparinized glass capillary tube. Determinations of pH, PCO_2, PO_2 and base excess are carried out immediately with the use of appropriate microelectrodes. After collection of the sample the incision site is compressed with a dry cotton swab for a few minutes to ensure hemostasis.

The reliability of capillary blood in assessment of the acid-base state of the fetus has been established by the fact that, in man, a high correlation was demonstrated between the pH of fetal capillary blood taken immediately before delivery and the pH of umbilical vein and umbilical artery blood obtained at the time of delivery, indicating that even in the second stage of labor blood flow through the fetal scalp is not sufficiently impaired to alter pH significantly. However, the formation of a caput succedaneum as a result of severe head compression may be associated with an abnormally low pH of blood in the scalp capillaries, due to local stasis.

Studies based on serial fetal blood sampling confirmed the decline in fetal blood pH and increase in PCO_2 occurring even during normal labor and delivery. A fetal capillary blood pH of 7.20 was defined as the lowest limit of normal, while values between 7.20 and 7.24 were considered "preacidotic." The validity of this classification was upheld by a good correlation between the pH of fetal samples collected shortly before delivery and Apgar scores at birth.

To distinguish acidosis originating in the mother from asphyxial acidosis in the fetus, one must compare the base deficit in the mother with that in the fetus. When the mother develops metabolic acidosis but placental function remains unimpaired, transfer of respiratory gases and of hydrogen ions proceeds normally and the difference between fetal and maternal base deficit (ΔBD) is small (mean 2.3 mEq/L). During fetal asphyxia associated with impairment of placental circulation there is accumulation of hydrogen ions in the fetal blood resulting in ΔBD in excess of 4.6 mEq/L.

BIOPHYSICAL FETAL MONITORING

Biophysical monitoring provides the physician with a continuous source of data relating to the fetus. A fetal monitor is a two-channel recorder of instantaneous fetal heart rate (FHR), along with associated uterine activity, both sets of data being necessary for the proper evaluation of labor. Depending on the method of obtaining fetal data, biophysical fetal monitoring can be characterized as direct or indirect.

Direct fetal monitoring

This type of surveillance is the most reliable because the fetal signal for the computation of instantaneous heart rate is obtained from an electrode attached to the fetal scalp. Intrauterine pressure is recorded continuously by a strain gauge, attached to a small catheter inserted transcervically into the amniotic cavity. This system provides accurate and quantitative information on frequency, duration, and intensity of contractions. However, it requires that the membranes be ruptured, cervical dilatation be at least 1.5 cm, and that the presenting part be dipping into the true pelvis. This type of direct monitoring is obviously limited to the true intrapartum period.

Indirect fetal monitoring

The indirect form of fetal surveillance relies on data obtained from transducers applied to the maternal abdomen overlying the gravid uterus. The following three systems are used to obtain FHR recordings: electro-, phono-, and ultrasound cardiography. Problems of separating fetal and maternal electrocardiographic complexes recorded from the maternal abdominal wall limit the applicability of the first approach. The use of a microphone is also limited because of a poor noise-to-signal ratio, particularly during uterine contractions. Thus, the most consistent method of obtaining fetal data from the maternal abdomen is by means of ultrasound cardiography.

Recording of uterine activity by the indirect system is obtained from a tocodynamometer, applied to the maternal abdomen, and triggered by the changing shape of the uterus during the contraction. Data thus obtained are quantitative only in respect to the frequency of contractions. The indirect method has the distinct advantages of simplicity and noninvasiveness.

Fetal well-being is determined by interpretation of the recordings, taking into consideration the following variables: (1) absolute heart rate, (2) beat-to-beat variability, (3) periodic patterns, and (4) uterine activity.

Rate. Normally it varies between 120 and 160 beats per minute. Persistently elevated rates may be associated with chronic fetal distress, maternal fever, and administration of drugs such as atropine. Abnormally low rates may be encountered in fetuses with congenital heart block.

Beat-to-beat variability. The fetal heart rate is under the control of the cerebral centers, reflexes and the integrated parasympathetic and sympathetic nervous system. When these divisions of the nervous system are functioning normally, variability will also be normal and the fetus is uniformly in good condition. Conversely, depression or damage of the fetal nervous system may result in minimal to absent variabilitity, which frequently occurs as the manifestation of fetal hypoxia or drug effect. Drugs most frequently associated with this phenomenon are: diazepam, local anesthetics, narcotics and barbiturates. Studies comparing beat-to-beat variability with fetal acid-base analysis indicate a good correlation between the two parameters.

Periodic patterns. Transient alterations of fetal heart rate associated with a contraction are called accelerations or decelerations, and are generally known as "periodic" patterns. These should be distinguished from baseline tachy- and bradycardia, which are deviations from the normal heart rate (120 - 160/min) occurring between uterine contractions.

Early deceleration. This uniform wavelike deceleration or slowing of the fetal heart rate starts with the onset of contraction, reaches its lowest point at the acme, and returns to baseline level at the termination of the contraction. The FHR usually does not fall below 100 beats per minute. This deceleration is thought to be caused by vagal stimulation secondary to compression of the head. It is not ameliorated by increasing fetal oxygenation, but is blocked by the administration of atropine. Most importantly, this pattern is not associated with deterioration of fetal acid-base status or with poor neonatal outcome.

Late deceleration. This is a uniform wave-like slowing the heart rate, the onset of deceleration being apparent after the onset of contraction. The slowest rate is reached after the acme of contraction, and FHR returns to baseline after the contraction has terminated. The etiology of this pattern is thought to be myocardial hypoxia resulting from uteroplacental insufficiency. The pattern of late deceleration can be corrected by improving fetal oxygenation. If this pattern is repetitive, continuous, and progressive in severity, there is a very significant correlation with a deteriorating fetal acid-base status.

Variable deceleration. This is the most common periodic pattern observed in the intrapartum period. As the term indicates, it is variable in shape and onset. Almost uniformly the FHR falls below 100 beats per minute. It is thought to be caused by umbilical cord compression and the resulting cardiovascular reflexes in the fetus. Administration of oxygen to the mother is without effect. If cord compression becomes more severe, prolonged and repetitive, fetal acidosis may develop.

Fetal scalp sampling was introduced in our institution in 1963, and was followed in 1969 by the adoption of biophysical monitoring. The two approaches to intrapartum fetal surveillance were integrated, and the following general guidelines for management have evolved:

1. In high-risk pregnancies, maternal and fetal pH and blood gases should be determined, whenever possible, before instituting biophysical monitoring.

2. All patients should be monitored by direct techniques as soon as possible.

3. In the face of a mixed pattern, the most ominous pattern should indicate the course of action.

4. When loss of beat-to-beat variability cannot be explained by the prior administration of a drug and persists for more than 30 - 45 minutes, a sample of fetal blood should be collected for acid-base determinations.

5. When repetitive late decelerations are detected, the following procedures should be initiated: (a) stop oxytocin if it is being infused; (b) administer oxygen at 6 - 7 liters per minute by a tight-fitting face mask; (c) correct hypotension, if present, by alteration in maternal position, administration of a vasopressor (e.g., ephedrine, 15 - 25 mg, iv), or expansion of intravascular fluid volume (e.g., lactated Ringer's solution, 500 - 1000 ml, iv); (d) collect free-flowing maternal venous and fetal capillary blood samples for acid-base determinations.

REFERENCES

1. Adamsons K, Beard RW, Bowe ET, et al: Standard practices at Sloane Hospital. Fetal blood sampling. Bull Sloane Hosp Women 13:11-15, 1967
2. Bowe ET, Beard RW, Finster M, et al: Reliability of fetal blood sampling. Am J Obstet Gynecol 107:279-287, 1970
3. Hon EH: 1968. An Atlas of Fetal Heart Patterns. New Haven, Conn, Harty Press.
4. Schifrin BS, Dame L: Fetal heart rate patterns, prediction of Apgar score. JAMA 219:1322-1325, 1972
5. Finster M, Petrie RH: Monitoring of the fetus. Anesthesiology 45:198-215, 1976

ARE INHALATION ANESTHETICS BETTER THAN INJECTABLE ANESTHETICS FOR CORONARY ARTERY SURGERY?

CASEY D. BLITT, M.D.

Historically, narcotic-oxygen anesthesia pioneered in Boston. This anesthetic (morphine-oxygen) was tailored for the severely-compromised cardiac patient with long-standing valvular heart disease. Patients had poorly-functioning myocardia with congestive heart failure, cardiomegaly and markedly altered chamber pressures and, in general, little cardiac reserve. It was found that these patients could be anesthetized with morphine and oxygen with minimal changes in cardiovascular variables.

Myocardial revascularization (CABG or"bypass") is frequently performed on patients with excellent myocardial function. Certainly a number of these patients may have poor myocardial reserve but we are routinely being presented with coronary artery disease patients who are not suffereing from a myriad of cardiac complications. These patients are not cardiac cripples, and are in reasonably good health. These patients are also, particularly from a physiologic standpoint, younger in years than patients having valvular surgery.

Thus, for the compromised cardiac patient with limited cardiac reserve, narcotic-oxygen anesthesia would appear to be an excellent choice. In fact, fentanyl is probably an even better drug than morphine for these valve-replacement patients.

The relatively healthy patient having saphenous vein coronary artery bypass grafting, because of one or more high-grade lesions in the coronary arteries, is a different situation. Is high dose, narcotic-oxygen better or are the inhalation anesthetic agents better for this patient? Inhalation anesthesia has some noteworthy advantages in these patients. They are:

1. The patient is anesthetized
2. Better minute-to-minute control of anesthetic depth is achieved
3. The sympathetic nervous system is blunted
4. There is a rapid termination of effect

Add to these criteria the limitations on narcotic anesthesia such as awareness and recall, chest wall rigidity, tachycardia, hypertension, nausea, and apnea and one would initially come to the conclusion that inhalation anesthesia is better than injectable anesthesia for coronary artery bypass surgery.

The answer is not that simple. Patients with poorly-functioning hearts, with poor ejection fractions, and elevated left ventricular end diastolic pressures will probably do better with the injectable agents. The healthy patient with good myocardial function may be more easily managed with inhalation agents. Halothane, enflurane, and isoflurane all have their good points for these patients. Halothane is the most arrhythmogenic and is the least potent peripheral vasodilator and depresses contractility the most of the three volatile agents. Enflurane is intermediate in all regards, and isoflurane depresses contractility the least, causes the most peripheral vasodilatation and along with enflurane is less arrhythmogenic than halothane.

Large dose narcotic (fentanyl) as a sole anesthetic has been shown to produce minimal changes in cardiovascular dynamics in patients with coronary artery disease. This effect is dose-dependent, however, and the appropriate point on the dose-response curve for any given patient must be found. A recent report concluded that "large doses of fentanyl as a sole anesthetic produce incomplete anesthesia and fail to protect the myocardium from ischemia due to noxious stimuli during coronary artery surgery."

In defense of injectable agents, they are not solely limited to large dose narcotics and some of the drawbacks of the narcotic-oxygen technique can be eliminated using additional injectable agents.

To attempt to answer the question originally asked, it would appear that injectable anesthetics confer a more stable cardiovascular state in patients with poor preoperative cardiac function. A <u>combination</u> of inhalation and injectable agents in patients with good myocardial function allows achievement of a salubrious balance between myocardial oxygen consumption and demand, provides an adequate anesthetic state, and is probably superior to narcotic-oxygen alone in this group of patients. In particular, a combination of isoflurane and fentanyl has worked remarkably well in our experience.

References

1. Stanley TH, Philbin DM, Coggins CH: Fentanyl-oxygen anesthesia for coronary artery surgery: cardiovascular and antidiuretic hormone responses. Can Anaesth Soc J 26:168-172, 1979.

2. Stanley TH, Berman L, Green O, et al: Plasma catecholamine and cortisol responses to fentanyl-oxygen anesthesia for coronary artery operations. Anesthesiology 53:250-254, 1980.

3. Waller JL, Hug CC, Nagle DM, et al: Fentanyl/oxygen anesthesia in coronary bypass surgery. Anesthesia & Analgesia (Cleve) 59:562-563, 1980.

4. Conahan TJ: Coronary artery disease -- special anesthetic considerations. in Cardiac Anesthesia. edited by TJ Conahan, III, M.D. Addison-Wesley, 1982.

5. Sonntag H, Larsen R, Hilfiker O, et al: Myocardial blood flow and oxygen consumption during high-dose fentanyl anesthesia in patients with coronary artery disease. Anesthesiology 56:417-422, 1982.

CONTINUOUS INFUSION OF INTRAVENOUS ANESTHETICS: AUTOMATED IV ANESTHESIA, A RATIONAL METHOD OF DRUG ADMINISTRATION

J.G. REVES, ERNEST R. GREENE, JR., THOMAS N. MACKRELL

There are four methods for intravenous (IV) anesthetic drug administration:

1. Intermittent without feedback
2. Intermittent with feedback
3. Continuous infusion without feedback
4. Continuous infusion with feedback.

The term feedback refers to information regarding the therapeutic effect of the administered drug. With anesthetic drugs, feedback may be the EEG to determine degree of CNS effect or electromyogram to monitor neuromuscular blockade. These are pharmacodynamic feedback systems. Most anesthetic courses involving intravenous drugs are conducted by intermittent infusion without feedback. Repeat doses of hypnotics (like thiopental or diazepam) are administered if the patient shows signs of awakening ("light anesthesia"). Analgesic compounds (like morphine, fentanyl, etc.) are administered when signs of activation of the sympathetic nervous system appear (increases of heart rate, blood pressure and lacrimation).

In Fig. 1, a drug level time course is presented. This is an idealized conceptualization in which administration of an IV drug immediately attains the therapeutic blood level, the blood level is maintained there, and with cessation of surgery the drug level abruptly drops below threshold. This time course is idealized and there are a number of unrealistic aspects: 1) it is impossible to know the threshold therapeutic level for each individual; 2) the therapeutic level will vary as the particular stress changes during the course of anesthesia and operation; 3) it is very difficult to have little or no overshoot in first attaining a desired blood level; and 4) very few drugs are biotransformed (metabolized) so rapidly that blood clearance drops off as precipitously as shown in Fig. 1.

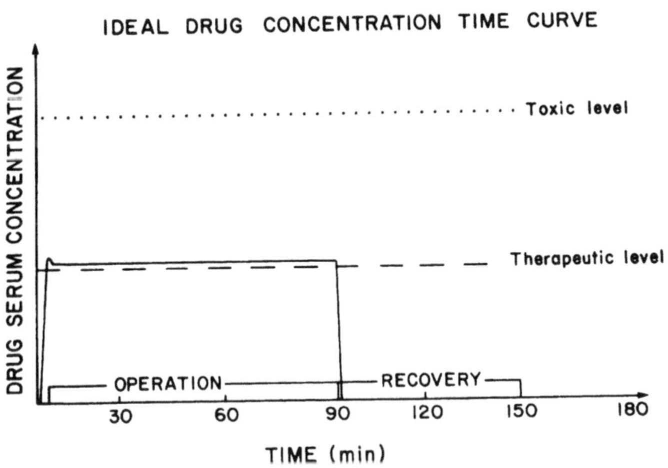

FIGURE 1.

Despite limitations of the idealized drug plasma time course, concepts in Fig. 1 represent a framework from which discussion of IV drug administration may be discussed. The actual practice of IV drug administration involves, in most cases, the intermittent administration of a drug whose elimination half-life exceeds the interval within which it is repeatedly administered. Drug accumulation (Fig. 2) results from repeat injections of a drug at intervals shorter than the elimination half-life (1). Thus during a case of multiple IV bolus administrations of IV drugs (e.g. fentanyl, diazepam, etc.) the plasma level of these drugs will rise, and presumably the action will be prolonged. If as in Fig. 2, a last administration is given to facilitate skin closure the highest drug levels will occur at end of operation causing a prolonged recovery. This contrasts markedly to the ideal drug time course in Fig. 1.

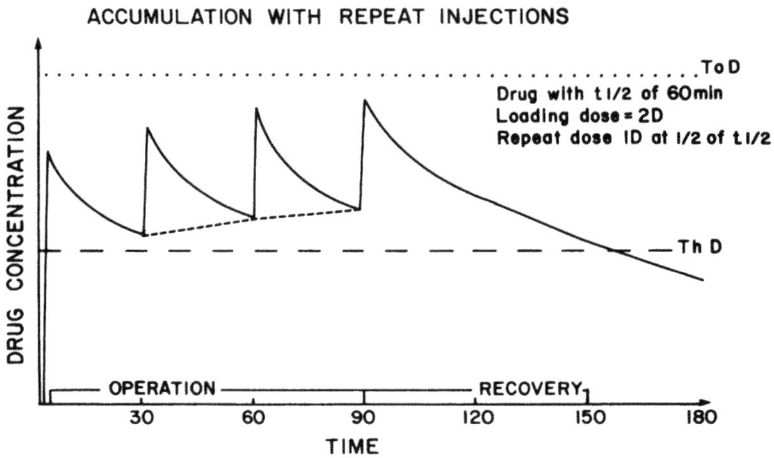

FIGURE 2.

An alternative method to intermittent drug administration is continuous infusion. Infusions can be designed to establish and maintain relatively constant blood levels just above the threshold value and well below a toxic level (Fig. 3). At the conclusion of surgery the drug infusion is discontinued with a prompt decrease in drug blood level. The best infusion method involves a closed-loop computer-assisted pharmacodynamic feedback system. There exists a hierarchy of computer involvement in the infusion of drugs: 1) manual-computer assisted, 2) programmed infusion without feedback, 3) programmed infusion with feedback, and 4) automatic control. At UAB, Dr. Louis Sheppard and coworkers have done this with the vasodilator, sodium nitroprusside, (2,3) to control mean arterial blood pressure and with the muscle relaxant, succinylcholine, to control the thenar electromyogram (4). A closed loop infusion of thiopental has been accomplished in rabbits utilizing spectral analysis of the EEG (5), but this technic has not been used successfully in man. Unfortunately, continuous administration of most anesthetic drugs cannot be governed by easily measured end-points since the pharmacodynamic effects are either not known or are not easily measured. Therefore, continuous administration is done without feedback or "blindly" (i.e. without the guidance provided by precise pharmacodynamic information regarding drug effects).

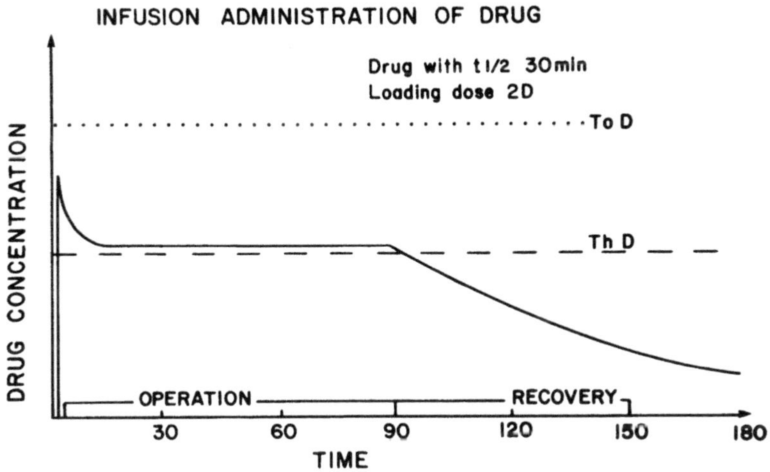

FIGURE 3.

A more rational method for infusion of anesthetic drugs may be based on knowledge of the particular drug's kinetics. This has been done with fentanyl (6) and can be done with any drug. This method allows the physician to administer IV anesthetics continuously to maintain predetermined therapeutic drug levels based upon pharmacokinetic data obtained from other patients. To facilitate and improve this type of infusion, we propose an automated method of IV drug infusion. One needs only the availability of reliable pharmacokinetic data and programmable infusion pumps to accomplish automated infusion. This information and equipment is currently available and easily assembled for clinical use. (See appendix.)

The choice of drug for use with a continuous infusion is important. The most desirable drug for continuous infusion without feedback is a drug with a large safety margin. Drugs with a large safety margin (Fig. 4A) produce the therapeutic effect at blood levels significantly lower than the blood levels which produce toxic effects. Examples of intravenous anesthetic drugs with large safety margins are fentanyl and ketamine. Drugs with a narrow margin of safety have an overlap of therapeutic and toxic drug blood levels (Fig. 4B). Thiopental is an example of intravenous drug which has a relatively narrow margin of safety, and although it has been used perhaps the most of any IV drug for infusion, it is not the best choice. Drugs with rapid plasma clearance are also theoretically better for infusion administration should overdosage be administered.

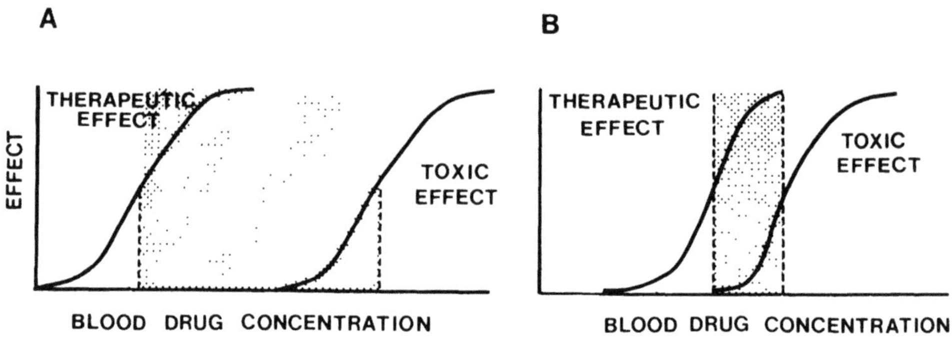

FIGURE 4.

The prospect of continuous infusions of intravenous drugs for use in balanced anesthesia is exciting since it permits tighter control of anesthetic administration than the usual intermittent method. However, there are limitations to this concept that must be considered when developing the infusion models. Some of these considerations include: 1) can kinetic data from some patients be applied to other patients with reasonable (and safe) predictability? 2) do drug plasma levels reflect drug receptor activity? 3) what if a drug produces acute tolerance or tachyphylaxis? 4) what about drug-drug interaction, for example, one drug displacing protein binding of another resulting in the second drug's increased effective concentration? 5) what if the case is prolonged, resulting in administration of doses that create zero-order kinetic clearance rates and invalidating the prediction of arousal time based on first-order kinetics? 6) are there acute changes in physiology, for example, changes in cardiac output or blood volume that can change the pharmacokinetic profile of the drugs? 7) does the modeling consider the appearance of a pharmacologically active metabolite, for example, desmethyl diazepam from diazepam? Future research will answer many of these questions (and probably raise many more).

We believe that the computer-assisted infusion of an intravenous anesthetic drug based on its pharmacokinetic properties is superior to either continuous or intermittent infusion without feedback. We are in the process of testing this hypothesis at UAB. In practice, the computer-assisted infusion designed to maintain a constant intravenous drug level may be likened to the administration of inhalation drugs which may also be kept at desired blood (end-tidal) levels. The development of appropriately programmed microprocessors and automated drug infusion pumps will allow the anesthesiologist to "dial in" his intravenous drugs as he currently does his inhalation drug. It is possible to include pharmacokinetic data in the memory of a small microprocessor for many intravenous anesthetics and to change from one drug to another with minimal time and effort. In the near future, we believe such computers and pumps will become a standard accessory for the anesthesia machine. We further propose that this form of automated infusion is the most rational of the currently available modes of administration of intravenous drugs.

APPENDIX

Attempts to use a steady infusion of drug by a syringe pump are usually not practical as the time to reach reasonable blood levels is excessive. The combination of an initial loading bolus dose to approximate quickly the desired level together with a steady infusion to offset elimination is only partially successful in maintaining a constant plasma level. The problem is that aside from elimination there is a significant time-dependent redistribution to peripheral compartments from the central compartment, of which plasma is one component. Following a loading dose, the infusion rate or drugs should not be constant. Rather it must change continuously as a function of time in a predetermined manner to keep the central concentration constant.

As an example, consider the new narcotic, sufentanil, to be kept at a therapeutic level of 1 ng/ml plasma concentration. Pharmacokinetic data for a 3 compartment model are available (7).

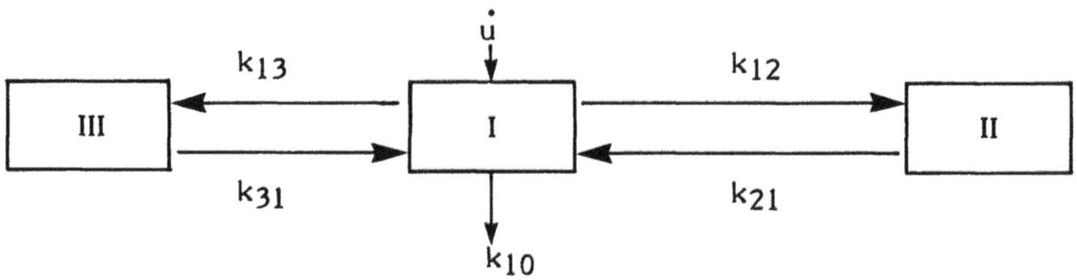

Here k_{12} refers to the first order rate constant for the transfer of drug from compartment 1 to compartment 2 and so forth. k_{10} is the rate constant for elimination from the central compartment and $\dot{u}$ is the rate of infusion of fresh drug. It has been found that:

$k_{10} = 8.73\ \text{hr}^{-1}$, $k_{12} = 40.19\ \text{hr}^{-1}$, $k_{13} = 11.57\ \text{hr}^{-1}$, $k_{21} = 16.74\ \text{hr}^{-1}$,
$k_{31} = 0.80\ \text{hr}^{-1}$.

The volume of compartment I, the central compartment, is $V_c = 0.104$ liter/kg body weight, W.

In each of the 3 compartments the rate of accumulation of drug equals the rate of input minus the rate of output of drug. In terms of differential equations for each compartment one has

$$\dot{C}_1 = -(k_{10} + k_{12} + k_{13})\, C_1 + k_{21}\, C_2 + k_{31}\, C_3 + \dot{u}/V_c$$
$$\dot{C}_2 = k_{12}\, C_1 - k_{21}\, C_2$$
$$\dot{C}_3 = k_{13}\, C_1 - k_{31}\, C_3$$

Here, for example, C_i is the concentration in compartment i and $\dot{C}_i$ is the rate of change of this concentration.

At time t = 0 there is no drug in compartments 2 and 3 so $C_2(0) = C_3(0) = 0$. The initial concentration in compartment 1 is $C_1(0)$ which is to be held constant for all times $t \geq 0$. The rate of infusion $\dot{u}(t)$ is to be determined such that $C_1(t) = C_1(0)$ for $t \geq 0$.

The solution to the set of differential equations with the specified initial conditions at t = 0 yields $\dot{u}(t)$, the desired rate of infusion to keep C_1 constant:

$$\dot{u}(t) = V_c\, C_1(0)\, (k_{10} + k_{12}\, e^{-k_{21}t} + k_{13}\, e^{-k_{31}t})$$

Note that the product $V_c\, C_1(0)$ equals the total mass of drug present in the central compartment. This is given as a single bolus, the loading dose, at time t = 0.

For the specific case of sufentanil, for $C_1(0)$ = 1 ng/ml and a patient of mass W kg this becomes

$$\dot{u}(t) = (104)(W)\, (0.1455 + 0.6698\, e^{-0.279t} + 0.1928\, e^{-.01333t})$$

In this expression if t is measured in minutes and W in kg, then $\dot{u}(t)$ will be given in terms of ng/min.

This expression can be programmed so that at each instant t the infusion pump delivers the specified infusion rate of drug by changing the rate of advancement of the pump's drive mechanism.

Acknowledgment

The authors wish to thank Dr. Louis Sheppard for his pioneering concepts and stimulation, Gilbert Ritchie for his assistance in solving our research problems, and Dr. Igor Kissin for his clear thinking regarding this project. We also acknowledge the clnical work with the automated control of muscle relaxation conducted by our colleague, Dr. John Ebert.

REFERENCES

1. Greenblatt DJ, Koch-Weser J. Clinical pharmacokinetics. N Engl J Med 1975;293:702-705.
2. Sheppard LC. Computer control of the infusion of vasoactive drugs. Ann Biomed Eng 1980;8:431-444.
3. Reves JG, Sheppard LC, Wallach R, et al. Therapeutic uses of sodium nitroprusside and an automated method of administration. International Anesthesiology Clinics 1978;16:51-88.
4. Ritchie GR, Ebert JP, Jannett TC, et al. A system for automatic control of muscle relaxation in surgical patients. (Unpublished).
5. Cosgrove RJ, Smolen VF. Systems for automatic feedback-controlled administration of drugs: analog and digital optimal-adaptive control of thiopental anesthesia. Proceeding of the San Diego Biomedical Symposium, North Hollywood, Western Periodicals, 1978:261-275.
6. Hengstmann JH, Stoeckel H, Schuttler J. Infusion model for fentanyl based on pharmacokinetic analysis. Br J Anaesth 1980;52:1021-1025.
7. Bovill JG, Sebel PS, Blackburn CL, et al. The pharmacokinetics of sufentanil in surgical patients. Janssen Pharmaceutica. (Unpublished).